AACN MISSION

AACN drives excellence in acute and critical care for nurses, patients and families.

AACN VISION

AACN is dedicated to creating a health care system driven by the needs of patients and families where acute and critical care nurses make their optimal contribution.

AACN CORE VALUES

As AACN works to promote its mission and vision, it is guided by values that are rooted in, and arise from, the Association's rich history, traditions and culture. Our values are the foundation upon which we build our relentless pursuit of excellence. AACN's members, volunteers and staff will honor the following:

- **Integrity** – We demonstrate sound judgment, ethical behavior and accountability in all we do.
- **Inclusion** – We cultivate an inclusive and equitable culture, where everyone contributes their unique strengths and perspectives.
- **Transformation** – We drive change and innovation to positively impact the health care system and improve the lives of patients, families and nurses.
- **Leadership** – We advocate and influence to achieve optimal outcomes and healthy work environments.
- **Relationships** – We collaborate and advance partnerships, honoring each individual to strengthen the collective.

AMERICAN ASSOCIATION of CRITICAL-CARE NURSES

AACN SCOPE AND STANDARDS FOR

Progressive Care Nursing Practice

2025

AMERICAN ASSOCIATION of CRITICAL-CARE NURSES

Editors:
Julie Miller, BSN, RN, CCRN
Sarah Wells, MSN, RN, CEN, CNL

Consulting Editor:
Judy Wilkin

Art Direction:
Michi Turner

An AACN Critical Care Publication
American Association of Critical-Care Nurses
27071 Aliso Creek Road
Aliso Viejo, CA 92656
Telephone: (800) 899-AACN
E-mail: info@aacn.org

ISBN 978-0-945812-25-8
AACN Product #130350

Printed in the USA

TABLE OF CONTENTS

ACKNOWLEDGMENTS

AACN Scope and Standards for Progressive Care Nursing Practice

Task Force Members

Anna Alder, DNP, RN, CCRN, NPD-BC – Chair
Kirsten Skillings, MA, APRN, CCRN, CCNS – AACN Board of Directors Liaison
Sara Knippa, MS, RN, ACCNS-AG, CCRN, PCCN – AACN Board of Directors Liaison
Jen Cousar, MSN, RN, PCCN, CCRN, CMSRN
Annie Guan, MSN, APRN, AGACNP-BC, PCCN, CV-BC
Amy Hemmer, MSN, RN, PCCN, HN-BC, CV-BC
Tristen Killen, MSN, RN, CCRN
Emily Schmitz, BSN, RN, PCCN
Tao Zheng, MN, RN, CCRN-CSC-CMC, CHFN, PCCN

Task Force AACN National Office Staff Liaisons

Julie Miller, BSN, RN, CCRN – Clinical Practice Specialist
Sarah Wells, MSN, RN, CEN, CNL – Clinical Practice Specialist

Invited Guests

Carol Bickford, PhD, RN-BC, CPHIMS, FHIMSS, FAAN
 Senior Policy Advisor, Department of Nursing Practice & Work Environment – American Nurses Association
Rebecca Callahan, BSN, RN, CMSRN, Academy of Medical-Surgical Nurses
Lindsey Green, DNP, MN, APRN-CNS, CCNS, RNC-NIC, Certification Practice Specialist
 Representing AACN Certification Corporation
Cindi Noe, MSN, RN, ICE-CCP, Certification Practice Specialist
 Representing AACN Certification Corporation
Rocio Sanchez, BSN, RN, PCCN, National Association of Hispanic Nurses
Tiffany Simon, MSN, RN, CCRN, Project Austin, Internal Affairs Manager Care Coordination – Society of Pediatric Nurses

A special acknowledgement is given to the organizations that supported the participation of members of the American Association of Critical-Care Nurses (AACN) and the representatives of other organizations who served on the task force for *AACN Scope and Standards for Progressive Care Nursing Practice.*

We are also indebted to the practicing nurses and faculty who provided thoughtful review and comments for this document throughout the period of public comment.

We are grateful for the dedication of everyone who helped research, write and review AACN Scope and Standards for Progressive Care Nursing Practice.

PURPOSE OF THIS DOCUMENT

Changes in health equity, diversity and inclusion, scientific knowledge, technology development, data collection and management, nursing workforce and staffing standards, health care reimbursement, and issues related to an aging society continue to drive the roles and responsibilities of nurses at all levels. The purpose of *AACN Scope and Standards for Progressive Care Nursing Practice*, 1st edition, is to describe the practice of nurses providing care to acutely ill patients in progressive care within the age parameters for which these nurses were educated — neonatal, pediatric, adult, and geriatric.

This document is intended for use by those involved in progressive care nursing, including students, faculty, nurses in practice, members of the interprofessional team, and other nursing colleagues. In addition, administrators, boards of nursing, policymakers, and insurers will benefit from the descriptions and accountabilities of progressive care registered nurses (RNs).

Progressive care nurses provide direct care or influence care for acutely ill patients who are moderately stable with an elevated risk for instability. These patients require a high intensity of care and vigilance.[1]

Progressive care nurses provide direct care based on the needs of patients. These patients are typically in areas such as telemetry, stepdown, intermediate, adaptable acuity, progressive care units (PCUs), emergency departments, and long-term acute care hospitals. These locations can include virtual nursing support where nurses monitor acutely ill patients from remote locations.[2]

The authors and contributors have attempted to describe the most current functions of the role in a manner consistent with nursing education and training, as well as licensure and certification, recognizing variations in scope of practice based on state regulations and hospital policies. The role of progressive care nurses must continue to evolve within this framework based on the needs of patients, families, and society.

The purpose of this document is to describe the practice of nurses providing care to acutely ill patients in progressive care within the age parameters for which these nurses were educated.

DEFINITION AND ROLE OF SCOPE

Scope of practice defines the boundaries of the practitioner's license (ie, the procedures, nursing actions, and processes for which the practitioner has received the education, training, licensure, and, if required, certification to practice in the state where the nurse works).[3] The exception to state rules and regulations occurs in nurse licensure compact states and in federal jurisdictions such as the US Department of Veterans Affairs. Documents defining scope of practice should describe who, what, when, where, why, and how the RN functions in their role. A scope of practice document should allow for expansion and flexibility of the profession to meet the changing needs of patients, families, organizations, and society.[4]

DEFINITION AND ROLE OF STANDARDS

Standards are "authoritative statements that describe the level of care or performance common to the profession of nursing by which the quality of nursing practice can be judged."[4] AACN standards explain the roles and responsibilities that the profession and society expect progressive care RNs to fulfill.

Standards of clinical practice describe a competent level of nursing practice, while *standards of professional performance* address the professional activities and behaviors expected of progressive care RNs. All standards include performance expectations, or *competencies*, that describe how progressive care nurses may demonstrate competent practice and build on the American Nurses Association's (ANA's) document *Nursing: Scope and Standards of Practice*, 4th edition.[5]

It is expected that the standards describing clinical practice and professional performance will remain stable over time. Competencies must continue to evolve to keep pace with changes in health equity, scientific evidence, new technologies, information, and data collection and management, and the needs of patients, families, and the health care system.

FRAMEWORK FOR THIS DOCUMENT

Nursing Process

The nursing process is a systematic method to organize professional nursing practice using critical thinking and diagnostic reasoning skills. Steps in the nursing process are composed of assessment, diagnosis, outcomes identification, planning, implementation, and evaluation.[5] Each step is predicated on the accuracy of the previous step; however, the process is dynamic rather than linear. Ongoing assessment of patients and families; their responses to interventions described in the plan; critical review and evaluation of available outcome information; and a reformulation of diagnoses, interventions, and expected outcomes occur along a continuum of care. The AACN Healthy Work Environment standards of skilled communication and true collaboration[6] among members of the interprofessional team, patients, and families/caregivers are critical to achieve optimal and equitable outcomes.

AACN Synergy Model for Patient Care

The fundamental premise of the *AACN Synergy Model for Patient Care*[7] is that optimal outcomes for patients and families occur when patient characteristics drive nurse competencies. Patients differ in their capacity for health and vulnerability to illness based on 8 core characteristics. The skills and level of competency required by the nurse are driven by the patient's needs along the continuum of those core patient characteristics.[8] AACN and AACN Certification Corporation embrace this model as a viable framework for progressive and critical care nursing practice.[7]

The AACN Synergy Model focuses on knowing the patient and understanding the perspectives of the patient and family. It integrates all dimensions of a patient's health status: physical, social, psychological, and spiritual. It reflects patient-driven and patient- and family-centered care that requires building relationships and achieves synergy when a healing environment is created and sustained.[9] The AACN Synergy Model includes consideration for the environment and systems in which health care is delivered as important factors in supporting nursing practices that drive optimal outcomes. See the glossary for definitions of patient characteristics and nurse competencies.

AACN Competence Framework for Progressive and Critical Care: Initial Competency 2022

AACN Competence Framework for Progressive and Critical Care: Initial Competency 2022[10] outlines the importance of using a core set of knowledge, skills, and abilities (KSAs), as well as a broader set of competencies that encompass nurses' ability to respond to the spectrum of rapidly changing patient and family needs. AACN offers a suggested list of core content-validated KSAs for adult critical and progressive care and pediatric intensive care that can be customized to align with the primary patient population on a specific unit. In addition, AACN defines 8 broader competencies that are based on the AACN Synergy Model[7] to complement the core KSAs and demonstrate nurses' ability to effectively address the spectrum of patients' needs. AACN provides specific content-validated performance outcomes (POs) to accompany each of these 8 synergy nurse competencies (SNCs) to help assess nurses' progress toward each competency.[7]

AACN Standards for Appropriate Staffing in Adult Critical Care

AACN Standards for Appropriate Staffing in Adult Critical Care[11] recommends 7 staffing standards that improve processes for nurse staffing in adult critical care. Each standard includes actions, tools, resources, and exemplars and leverages the 6 AACN Healthy Work Environment standards. While foundational, *AACN Standards for Appropriate Staffing in Adult Critical Care*[11] must be combined with collaboration and a commitment to change from nurses, staff, and leaders. The standards are broad, and while originally written for adult critical care, they offer guidance that also may be applied to the progressive care setting. AACN plans to publish staffing standards for progressive care in 2025.

AACN Tele-critical Care Nursing Practice: An Expert Consensus Statement Supporting Acute, Progressive, and Critical Care 2022

AACN Tele-critical Care Nursing Practice: An Expert Consensus Statement Supporting Acute, Progressive, and Critical Care 2022[2] offers recommendations, clinical vignettes, and a framework to implement, assess, and improve evolving practices in the progressive care space. The document provides a comprehensive, patient-centric approach that incorporates essential tele-critical care elements and adaptations for the rapidly evolving world of virtual nursing. It also reflects current evidence to support optimal progressive care nursing practice.

AACN Standards for Establishing and Sustaining Healthy Work Environments

AACN Standards for Establishing and Sustaining Healthy Work Environments[6] provides a framework to create an environment where progressive care nurses, patients, families, and the interprofessional team work together to meet the goals of care. The 6 standards (skilled communication, true collaboration, effective decision making, appropriate staffing, meaningful recognition, and authentic leadership), all essential components of a healthy work environment, support nurses as part of the interprofessional team to coordinate optimal care delivery for the benefit of the patient, all team members, and the organization.[6]

ANA's Code of Ethics for Nurses with Interpretive Statements

All nurses have an ethical obligation to themselves, patients and families, and society, as described in ANA's *Code of Ethics.*[12] Part of the framework for the AACN scope and standards is to remind nurses of this continual obligation. It is an essential document within the context of progressive care, given the highly stressful situations that occur in this environment that can lead to moral, psychological, and physical distress for nurses.

AACN Scope and Standards for Progressive and Critical Care Nursing Practice

In 2019, *AACN Scope and Standards for Progressive and Critical Care Nursing Practice*[13] established how to describe and measure the expected level of practice and professional performance for RNs practicing in those care areas. With the expansion and evolution of the progressive care nursing specialty, the need for a dedicated scope and standards for progressive care nursing practice became evident. *AACN Scope and Standards for Progressive Care Nursing Practice* is built on the foundation provided by *AACN Scope and Standards for Progressive and Critical Care Nursing Practice*[14] and ANA's *Nursing: Scope and Standards of Practice*, 4th edition.[5]

Characteristics of Nursing Practice

The 3 characteristics of nursing practice are as follows:

- A link exists between the work environment and the RN's ability to practice.[6]
- Nursing practice is individualized to meet the unique needs of the patient or situation.[8]
- Nurses establish partnerships with the patient, family, support system, and other members of the interprofessional team.[5]

In addition to these characteristics and those in the AACN Synergy Model[7] and *AACN Competence Framework for Progressive and Critical Care: Initial Competency 2022,*[10] the Progressive Care Scope and Standards Task Force used the following assumptions in regard to progressive care nursing practice:

- *Wherever acutely ill patients receive care, nurses are required to have the competence to care for them.*[8] This statement rules out labeling progressive care nurses as those who work only in a traditional PCU. The boundaries of PCUs have expanded beyond traditional walls into environments such as other areas of the hospital, virtual units (eg, telehealth, virtual nursing), the community, and homes.
- *Nurses build their KSAs in a cumulative fashion, progressing from novices with basic competencies to expert practitioners.*[14] The time frame for building and integrating their abilities into clinical practice is usually different for each nurse, and not all nurses will reach an expert level of practice. The characteristics of competent nursing care reflect the integration of knowledge, skills, attitudes, and experience.
- *Nursing is a dynamic and cyclical process that is holistic in nature.* Nurses are continually collecting, analyzing, and interpreting information and data from multiple sources to critically evaluate and revise the plan of care.[5] Nurses realize that understanding the needs, values, beliefs, and attitudes of patients and their families or loved ones is integral to the success of the plan. They actively seek and share such information and then incorporate it into the plan, as needed.[5]

REFERENCES

1. AACN Certification Corporation. Practice analysis of the progressive care nurse. AACN Certification Corporation; 2023.

2. American Association of Critical-Care Nurses. *AACN Tele-critical Care Nursing Practice: An Expert Consensus Statement Supporting Acute, Progressive and Critical Care 2022.* American Association of Critical-Care Nurses; 2022. Accessed April 25, 2024. https://www.aacn.org/nursing-excellence/standards/aacn-tele-critical-care-nursing-consensus-statement

3. National Council of State Boards of Nursing. Nurse licensure compact. https://www.ncsbn.org/compacts.page

4. National Academies of Sciences, Engineering, and Medicine. *The Future of Nursing 2020-2030: Charting a Path to Achieve Health Equity.* The National Academies Press; 2021. doi:10.17226/25982

5. American Nurses Association. *Nursing: Scope and Standards of Practice.* 4th ed. American Nurses Association; 2021. Accessed April 29, 2024. https://www.nursingworld.org/nurses-books/nursing-scope-and-standards-of-practice-4th-edit/

6. Barden C, ed. *AACN Standards for Establishing and Sustaining Healthy Work Environments: A Journey to Excellence.* 2nd ed. American Association of Critical-Care Nurses; 2016. https://www.aacn.org/nursing-excellence/standards/aacn-standards-for-establishing-and-sustaining-healthy-work-environments

7. AACN Certification Corporation. AACN Synergy Model for Patient Care. Accessed August 13, 2024. http://www.aacn.org/wd/certifications/content/synmodel.pcms?menu=certification

8. Curley MAQ. *Synergy: The Unique Relationship Between Nurses and Patients.* Sigma Theta Tau International; 2007.

9. AACN Certification Corporation. *Certification Exam Policy Handbook.* American Association of Critical-Care Nurses; 2024. https://www.aacn.org/certification/preparation-tools-and-handbooks/handbooks-and-documents

10. *AACN Competence Framework for Progressive and Critical Care: Initial Competency 2022.* American Association of Critical-Care Nurses; 2022. https://www.aacn.org/nursing-excellence/standards/aacn-competence-framework-for-progressive-and-critical-care

11. Delgado SA, Good V, Barden C, Cassidy L, eds. *AACN Standards for Appropriate Staffing in Adult Critical Care.* American Association of Critical-Care Nurses; 2024. Accessed April 27, 2024. https://www.aacn.org/-/media/aacn-website/nursing-excellence/standards/aacn-standards-for-appropriate-staffing-in-adult-critical-care.pdf

12. American Nurses Association. *Code of Ethics for Nurses with Interpretive Statements.* Nursesbooks.org; 2015.

13. American Association of Critical-Care Nurses. *AACN Scope and Standards for Progressive and Critical Care Nursing Practice.* American Association of Critical-Care Nurses; 2019. Accessed May 5, 2024. https://www.aacn.org/-/media/aacn-website/nursing-excellence/standards/aacn-scope-and-standards-for-progressive-and-critical-care-nursing-practice.pdf

14. Benner P. *From Novice to Expert: Excellence and Power in Clinical Nursing Practice.* Addison-Wesley; 1984.

PROFESSIONAL TRENDS AND ISSUES

Post-pandemic issues central to nursing such as nurse-to-patient staffing; nurse well-being; the health of the work environment; safe, equitable and quality care; virtual and telehealth solutions, as well as health system concerns such as value-based purchasing (VBP), Hospital Consumer Assessment of Healthcare Providers and Systems (HCAHPS), and health care policies, affect the climate in which nurses work.[1] The challenge for nurses is to remain proactive leaders who adapt in response to the increasingly complex needs of patients, families, and work environments. The challenges to meeting these needs include the following:

- The ongoing nurse staffing crisis, turnover, and retirement of nurses
    - Nursing turnover continues to impact the ability to staff progressive care units safely. The highest rates for nursing turnover in 2023 were for nurses working in telemetry (115%), stepdown units (119%), and emergency services (112%). It is estimated that these units turn over their entire nursing staff in less than 4.5 years.[2] Nurses in their first year continue to have turnover rates of approximately 34%.[1] Turnover and retirement of nurses result in a significant loss of experience and knowledge, which is contributing to a widening experience-complexity gap.[3]
    - Opportunities are increasing for professional development beyond traditional roles in progressive care nursing. For example, transfers to critical care units, advanced practice and leadership positions, and the growth in virtual nurse opportunities draw nurses away from traditional roles as direct care progressive care nurses.
    - RN vacancy rates remain elevated at 9.9%, resulting in excess labor costs such as overtime, critical staffing pay, salary increases, and travel/agency usage. Elevated vacancy rates, along with difficulty recruiting RNs, indicate the staffing crisis will continue to impact hospitals.[2]
    - These issues are contributing to shortages of progressive care nursing personnel, resulting in a constant need to hire and educate progressive care nurses, and additional hospital costs.[2]
    - Nurses who remain in their jobs are facing increased workloads and job-related stress due to these issues.[4]
- An explosion of technology and medical advances, as well as regulatory changes, requires continual learning. These non-direct patient care tasks take time away from direct patient care.[5]
- Transitioning newly trained clinicians from education to practice was listed[5] as ECRI's number 1 patient safety concern for 2024. These nurses are welcome additions to unit staffing, but without sufficient preparation and support in acclimating them to nursing practice, they may not recognize deterioration in a patient's condition, delay rescuing patients from preventable harm, or cause direct patient harm.[5]

- Nurses new to progressive care may lack full knowledge and competencies for specialty practice, but they bring passion, engagement, and new perspectives. To successfully integrate novice nurses into practice, and to support professional growth and the development of knowledge and competence, a supportive, healthy work environment that provides the necessary resources and infrastructure is needed.[6]
- The health of the work environment declined during and immediately following the pandemic, with the largest decline occurring in the AACN standard for appropriate staffing. In some work environments, nurses are faced with incivility, bullying, and/or violence, including physical/psychological harm.[4] These situations create an unhealthy work environment where maintaining one's safety distracts from nursing care. Nurses who work in healthier work environments report less burnout, a lower intent to leave their organizations, and less job dissatisfaction.[4]
- Shortages of medications and supplies necessary to provide care contribute to the daily stress of the work environment.

The impact over time of these unresolved challenges also leads to stress in the work environment that may result in 1 or more issues. For example:

- Burnout Syndrome
    - Burnout syndrome adversely affects nurses' ability to care for patients due to feelings of emotional stress and job-related disillusionment, resulting in an inability to adapt to the work environment.[6]
- Moral Distress
    - Nurses are often presented with ethical challenges when faced with competing core values or commitments and diverse viewpoints on how to reconcile them, which may include the perception of inappropriate delivery of patient care.[7] In these situations, the nurse may know or think they know the correct action to take but are constrained from taking it. This situation may result in moral distress.[8]
- Compassion Fatigue
    - The emotional effect of being indirectly traumatized after helping someone who has experienced primary traumatic stress may result in loss of empathy and a gradual reduction in the ability to show compassion. Nurses who witness patients experiencing devastating illnesses or trauma may react by distancing themselves from their feelings, leading to a sense of helplessness and anger. Compassion fatigue is often linked to burnout.[8]
- Engagement in Profession
    - Nurses' engagement in the profession varies and affects their capability to manage work stressors. Their degree of engagement and the resilience to handle work stressors correlate highly to their intention to remain in their jobs.[9]

These issues may arise throughout nurses' careers. They affect nurses professionally and personally, and may negatively impact their ability to meet the needs of their patients. These situations may lead to nurses leaving the profession.[8]

Staffing to match the needs of the patient with the competencies of the nurse continues to be a topic of discussion among nursing professionals on how it can best be accomplished. Two critical elements specific to appropriate staffing declined significantly in *National Nurse Work Environments - October 2021: A Status Report*.[4] "RN staffing ensures the effective match between patient needs and nurse competencies" declined significantly from 2018 to 2021, and only 24% of participants reported having "the right number of RNs with the right knowledge and skills" more than 75% of the time or all of the time.[4]

In addition, nurses continue to focus on how their contribution to patient and quality outcomes affects the financial stability of the systems where they work. Nurses are engaged in and/or leading many quality-improvement initiatives that take them away from direct patient care. In many instances, this time away from patient care is recorded as nonproductive time. Yet many of these nurses indicate that these projects have a sustained financial savings for the health system.[10] Nonproductive time does not necessarily imply a lack of cost-effectiveness.[11] Evidence has demonstrated that investing in the engagement of frontline nurses in the leadership of quality-improvement initiatives leads to sustainable and scalable improvements with positive impacts on clinical, organizational, and financial outcomes. This outcome requires that nurses are afforded protected time away from direct care. It is time for a paradigm shift in thinking regarding nursing time spent on quality-improvement projects.[3]

Another influential trend that affects nurses is VBP. This trend and HCAHPS provide financial incentives to hospitals, physicians, and other health care providers to carry out quality improvements and achieve optimal outcomes for patients. The financial impact of this current focus is being felt across the health care continuum. Nurses play an integral role in improving patient/family satisfaction and patient outcomes, such as preventing falls and pressure injuries, and subsequently improving hospital fiscal outcomes.[10] Investing in appropriate nurse staffing leads to better outcomes and improved patient safety.[3]

Progressive care nurses also face workflow challenges, because the acuity and number of patients they treat may fluctuate throughout their shifts. Admissions and discharges increase nursing workloads and require a high level of diligence and attention to detail. In addition, nurses often are transferring out lower-acuity patients to admit higher-acuity patients. These factors and the number of patients a nurse may care for require a high degree of flexibility and redirection of available resources to meet the changing acuity, volume, and complexity. This churn in patient care workload can result in a complete turnover of a nurse's patient assignment in an 8- or 12-hour shift. For example, a PCU nurse may take an assignment of 3 patients at the beginning of the shift, but after all the admissions, discharges, and transfers in and out, the nurse has actually cared for 6 or more patients during that time frame.

Nurses' ability to adjust focus rapidly may be affected by this churn in patient care. Nursing care varies based on the acuity of each patient, and the needs of the patient must be matched to the competencies of the nurse.[12] Each nurse must develop the competencies to prioritize and treat patients, as well as manage changing workflows, based on the frequency of patient turnover. Nurses frequently report that documentation requirements take them away from direct patient care. The high frequency of patient turnover contributes to an increased documentation workload for nurses. This situation can result in less detailed documentation and handoff communication when nurses are faced with high patient turnover. Transitions of care and handoffs have been targeted as an area for improvement due to the risks for errors and patient harm.[13]

National initiatives that focus on improving the quality of nursing care, improving staffing,[3,14] reducing health care-acquired conditions and adverse events, and providing safe care to all who need it influence the composition of health care teams. A growing number of older adults seeking health care services are influencing not only the way that care is provided, but also the clinical education and preparation required of their providers. In addition, a growing number of patients have outlived what were once considered pediatric conditions without expected survival to adulthood.

In addition, health equity and its impact on patient outcomes is a leading issue in ensuring safe, equitable care. ANA's *Nursing Scope and Standards of Practice, Standard 9: Respectful and Equitable Practice* states that the RN practices with cultural humility and inclusiveness.[15] ANA's *Code of Ethics for Nurses* also focuses on nurses' commitment to social justice.[16] With commitment to these standards, nurses can reduce gaps in health outcomes and improve equity in health care. To be successful, nurses need to strengthen their knowledge and skill in applying principles of equity, diversity, and inclusion.[17]

Patients with complex medical and nursing problems and their families are demanding higher-quality and safer care, more attention to the patient's experience, and greater transparency in the health care system. The Patient-Centered Outcomes Research Institute (PCORI) funds studies that can help patients and those who care for them make better-informed health care choices.[18] Patients and their families are becoming more informed consumers of health care and are entering the health care system with a variety of perspectives shaped by their search for information.

Trends in the health care environment and societal changes also affect the required education and competencies of nurses caring for acutely ill patients. The increased emphasis on artificial intelligence; equity, diversity, and inclusion principles; genomics-based medicines; and alternative care models such as telehealth; as well as ongoing medical advances; impact the required KSAs and attitudes of health care providers. Nurses must have access to ongoing, high-quality continuing education to maintain the knowledge and skills necessary to provide the level of care their patients need.

Artificial intelligence algorithms to identify trends in a patient's condition and to assist with clinical decision support are available and being developed to reduce cognitive load for nurses and improve efficiency of care and patient safety.[19,20] Ever-increasing and complex clinical and information technology solutions require a level of technological acumen that can be difficult to incorporate into nurses' everyday work. Nurses are responsible for prioritizing patient care needs, material resources, time, and documentation, while remaining vigilant to care for the complex needs of patients and families.

The growth of telehealth, tele-critical care, and virtual nursing extends care beyond the traditional hospital walls to a virtual community and expands the interprofessional care team. These advances provide health care providers with the opportunity to collaborate with other care providers to supplement and expand their knowledge and skills while supporting patients and improving outcomes.[21] The competencies required to work and collaborate with providers of tele-critical care and virtual nursing support are not currently included in the nursing curriculum.

Technological advances allow the interprofessional team to sustain life almost indefinitely. Nurses attend to the needs of these patients while providing them and their families the information they require to weigh the benefits and risks of these life-sustaining treatments. The increased ability to extend life through technology has also created situations in which further care may not be beneficial, or goals of care may change. Nurses advocate for shared decision making in which patients and families have a full understanding of quality-of-life and end-of-life decisions. The need for nurses who are adept in managing ethical issues becomes ever more important. Skill in communicating with patients and families at the level of their understanding is critical. Development and maintenance of competent end-of-life care is an essential component in caring for acutely and critically ill patients in any environment.

Public health emergencies such as the COVID-19 pandemic and natural and environmental disasters demonstrate the need to have nurses who are prepared to respond and help treat affected individuals and communities. Preparation must include the KSAs to respond in a variety of roles, and nurses must have an awareness of the social determinants of health (SDOH) that may adversely affect the individuals in their care.[17]

A positive relationship exists between the health of the nursing work environment, job satisfaction, and intent to stay.[4] Physical and verbal abuse from patients, families, and interprofessional staff harm both the individual and the work environment. Respondents to *National Nurse Work Environments - October 2021: A Status Report* reported more than 216 767 incidents of verbal abuse, physical abuse, discrimination, and sexual harassment within the previous 12 months. The study reported the most frequent source of abuse was patients and families. Nearly one-half of respondents did not believe their facilities valued their safety and health.[4] Since nurse and patient outcomes are partially associated with work environments, more work needs to be done to ensure the health and safety of the nursing work environment.

The degree of nurses' professional and organizational engagement is directly correlated with quality care, the patient experience, and critical safety outcomes.[22] An analysis of data from a Press Ganey database estimates that clinical nurse engagement is slowly improving but continues to need attention to ensure nurses are satisfied with their work and remain employed. Disengaged staff results in increased likelihood for safety events, lower patient experience scores, and higher rates of burnout and turnover.[23] Nurses often must balance their individual and personal commitments with their engagement in the profession, resulting in issues with work-life balance. Varying levels of engagement also affect the health of the work environment. Strategies to support nurse engagement should address the following issues:

- Improving the health of the work environment results in nurses reporting less moral distress, improved quality of care, less intent to leave, and improved patient satisfaction.[4]
- Multiple generations of nurses in the workforce have different styles of engagement and communication that can create conflict in the workplace. Adaptability and focusing on the work environment, work-life balance, nurse well-being, and career growth are essential to improve engagement.[9] Better work-life balance has positive effects on patient safety and the work environment.[24]
- Using virtual care, technology, and social media solutions can help nurses develop creative ways to foster engagement in the profession.
- Lack of nurses' input at the highest levels of local, state, and national organizations must be addressed. The current Nurses on Boards Coalition initiative brings the unique perspectives of nurses to achieve their goals of improved health for patients and efficient and effective health care systems.[25]

Progressive care nurses are in demand and need to make their optimal contribution to patients and families. It is essential that each nurse understand the purpose, expectations, and boundaries inherent in the scope and standards of practice and professional performance to ensure their practice supports patients and families, professional values, and long-term engagement with the profession.

Progressive care nurses are in demand and need to make their optimal contribution to patients and families.

REFERENCES

1. American Organization for Nursing Leadership Foundation. *Nursing Leadership Insight Longitudinal Study.* American Organization for Nursing Leadership; 2024. Accessed May 14, 2024. https://www.aonl.org/resources/nursing-leadership-survey

2. NSI Nursing Solutions Inc. *2024 NSI National Health Care Retention & RN Staffing Report.* NSI Nursing Solutions Inc; 2024. Accessed May 4, 2024. https://www.nsinursingsolutions.com/Documents/Library/NSI_National_Health_Care_Retention_Report.pdf

3. American Association of Critical-Care Nurses. *AACN Standards for Appropriate Staffing in Adult Critical Care.* Accessed May 14, 2024. https://www.aacn.org/-/media/aacn-website/nursing-excellence/standards/aacn-standards-for-appropriate-staffing-in-adult-critical-care.pdf

4. Ulrich B, Cassidy L, Barden C, Varn-Davis N, Delgado SA. National nurse work environments - October 2021: a status report. *Crit Care Nurse.* 2022;42(5):58–70. Accessed May 14, 2024. https://doi.org/10.4037/ccn2022798

5. ECRI Institute. ECRI's top 10 patient safety concerns 2024. Accessed May 14, 2024. https://home.ecri.org/blogs/ecri-blog/ecri-s-top-10-patient-safety-concerns-for-2024

6. American Association of Critical-Care Nurses. *AACN Standards for Establishing and Sustaining Healthy Work Environments: A Journey to Excellence.* 2nd ed. Accessed May 14, 2024. https://www.aacn.org/-/media/aacn-website/nursing-excellence/standards/hwestandards.pdf

7. Rushton CH. Transforming moral suffering by cultivating moral resilience and ethical practice. *Am J Crit Care.* 2023;32(4):238-248. Accessed May 14, 2024. https://doi.org/10.4037/ajcc2023207

8. Moss M, Good VS, Gozal D, et al. An official Critical Care Societies collaborative statement: burnout syndrome in critical care health care professionals: a call for action. *Am J Crit Care.* 2016;25(4):368–376. https://qualitysafety.bmj.com/content/28/2/142

9. Wright M. Engagement matters: meeting the unique challenges of the healthcare workforce. Press Ganey; 2022. Accessed May 14, 2024. https://info.pressganey.com/press-ganey-blog-healthcare-experience-insights/engagement-matters-meeting-the-unique-challenges-of-the-healthcare-workforce

10. Lacey SR, Goodyear-Bruch C, Olney A, et al. Driving organizational change from the bedside: the AACN Clinical Scene Investigator Academy. *Crit Care Nurse.* 2017;37(4):e12–e25. https://aacnjournals.org/ccnonline/article/37/4/e12/3692/Driving-Organizational-Change-From-the-Bedside-The

11. Altman M, Rosa W. Redefining "time" to meet nursing's evolving demands. *Nurs Crit Care.* 2018;11(3):12–15. https://journals.lww.com/nursing/abstract/2016/03000/redefining__time__to_meet_nursing_s_evolving.16.aspx

12. American Association of Critical-Care Nurses. *AACN Competence Framework for Progressive and Critical Care: Initial Competency 2022.* Accessed May 14, 2024. https://www.aacn.org/nursing-excellence/standards/aacn-competence-framework-for-progressive-and-critical-care

13. Sehgal N. AHRQ Patient Safety Network. Perspectives on safety: handoffs and transitions. Accessed September 26, 20 24. https://psnet.ahrq.gov/perspective/handoffs-and-transitions

14. American Nurses Association. Safe staffing. Accessed May 14, 2024. https://www.nursingworld.org/practice-policy/nurse-staffing/

15. American Nurses Association. *Nursing: Scope and Standards of Practice.* 4th ed. American Nurses Association; 2021. Accessed May 15, 2024. https://www.nursingworld.org/nurses-books/nursing-scope-and-standards-of-practice-4th-edit/

16. American Nurses Association. *Code of Ethics for Nurses with Interpretive Statements.* Nursesbooks.org; 2015.

17. Flaubert JL, Le Menestrel S, Williams DR, et al, eds. *The Future of Nursing 2020-2030: Charting a Path to Achieve Health Equity.* National Academies Press; 2021. https://www.ncbi.nlm.nih.gov/books/NBK573904/

18. Patient-Centered Outcomes Research Institute. Accessed May 14, 2024. https://www.pcori.org

19. Rony MKK, Kayesh I, Bala SD, Akter F, Parvin MR. Artificial intelligence in future nursing care: exploring perspectives of nursing professionals - a descriptive qualitative study. *Heliyon*. 2024;10(4):e25718. doi:10.1016/j.heliyon.2024.e25718

20. Alderden JG, Johnny JD. Artificial intelligence and the critical care nurse. *Crit Care Nurse*. 2023;43(5):7–8. https://doi.org/10.4037/ccn2023755

21. American Association of Critical-Care Nurses. *AACN Tele-critical Care Nursing Practice: An Expert Consensus Statement Supporting Acute, Progressive and Critical Care 2022*. Accessed September 25, 2024. https://www.aacn.org/nursing-excellence/standards/aacn-tele-critical-care-nursing-consensus-statement

22. Waddoups J. Active nursing professional engagement. *Am Nurse*. 2022;17(7). Accessed May 14, 2024. https://www.myamericannurse.com/active-nursing-professional-engagement/

23. Schwartz SP, Adair KC, Bae J, et al. Work-life balance behaviours cluster in work settings and relate to burnout and safety culture: a cross-sectional survey analysis. *BMJ Qual Saf*. 2018;0:1–9.

24. Nurses on Boards Coalition. Accessed May 14, 2024. https://www.nursesonboardscoalition.org/

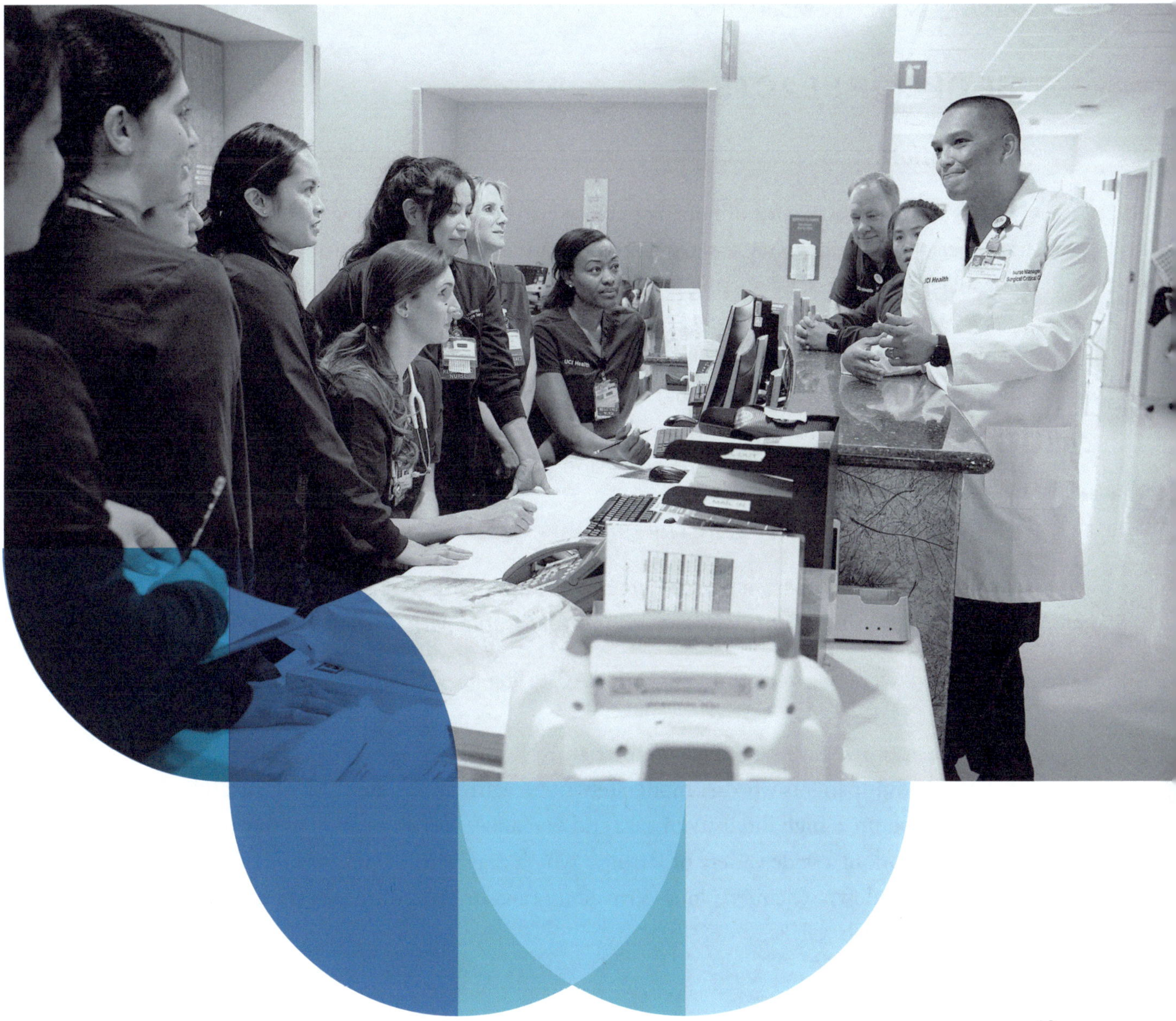

SCOPE OF PRACTICE FOR PROGRESSIVE CARE NURSING

INTRODUCTION

The delivery of quality care to acutely and critically ill and injured patients and their families is the primary goal of the American Association of Critical-Care Nurses (AACN), since its inception in 1969. The historical conceptualization of nursing delineates clinical practice dimensions according to the practitioner's role, the clinical setting, a patient's diagnosis, and a patient's physiologic and psychosocial systems. Today's changing health care calls for the complexities and needs of patients to drive the competencies of nurses and advanced nursing practice. These required competencies reflect the integration of knowledge, skills, and attitudes needed to meet the patients' needs as defined by the AACN Synergy Model.[1]

SCOPE OF PRACTICE

Foundation

ANA's scope and standards of nursing practice are the basis of nursing practice, providing a foundation for specialty practice. They serve as a template for delineating the distinguishing characteristics and complexities of specialty nursing practice. *AACN Scope and Standards for Progressive Care Nursing Practice* builds on ANA's *Nursing: Scope and Standards of Practice,* 4th edition[2] (2021) and does not replace it. Progressive care nurses are expected to practice in accordance with the competencies identified in both documents. Progressive care scope of practice incorporates the contributions and domains of nursing and specialty nursing practice. Although progressive care nursing is a distinct specialty, it is inseparable from the profession of nursing as a whole.

Definition: Progressive Care Nursing

AACN defines progressive care nursing as the specialty that provides care to or influences the care of acutely ill patients who are moderately stable with an elevated risk of instability.

Progressive Care Nurse Definition From AACN Practice Analysis for the Progressive Care Nurse Study of Practice[3]

- A progressive care nurse is either an RN or APRN who provides direct care for acutely ill adult patients who are moderately stable with an elevated risk of instability. These patients require a high intensity of care and vigilance. Nurses practicing in this specialty area may work in a wide variety of settings, which may include progressive care, intermediate care, stepdown, telemetry, long-term acute care, or procedure labs (radiology, electrophysiology, cath lab, GI).

- ◦ The focus of this definition on adults is because the practice analysis study for progressive care involves only nurses caring for the adult population requiring progressive care.

The Progressive Care Scope and Standards Task Force's discussion and review of the literature validate that progressive care nursing also encompasses the direct care of patients across the life span and is not limited to adults.

Progressive care nurses may be required to refine their assessment skills supported only by limited monitoring technology. Progressive care nurses include nurses working in tele-critical care/virtual nursing, monitoring acutely ill patients from a remote location.[3] As members of the profession, progressive care nurses are committed to protecting, maintaining, and optimizing the health of patients entrusted to their care. Progressive care nurses' unique challenge is to create safety and optimize outcomes for patients at an elevated risk for instability and their families.

The scope of practice for nursing care of patients of all ages encompasses the dynamic interaction of the patient and family, the nurse, and the environment where care is being provided, with a goal of ensuring optimal patient outcomes. Nurses recognize patients and families as the fundamental and central focus for the delivery of nursing care. A commitment to the vision of a patient- and family-centered health care system requires a holistic view of patients and families, as well as recognition of their multiple dimensions, including physical, psychological, emotional, spiritual and cultural needs, and social determinants of health. This commitment requires terms such as *care choices* and *family* to be defined from the patient's perspective.

The foundation of progressive care nursing practice is based on a body of specialized scientific knowledge, an ethical model for decision making, nurse/patient/system interrelatedness described in the AACN Synergy Model,[4] and a commitment to interprofessional collaboration. This foundation highlights the unique value nurses bring to caring for this patient population. Progressive care nurses rely on this foundation to:

- Ensure the delivery of safe, compassionate, holistic, and high-quality patient care.
- Provide for patient- and family-centered care, which has been described as an "approach to the planning, delivery, and evaluation of health care that is grounded in mutually beneficial partnerships among health care providers, patients, and families."[5]
- Restore, support, promote, rehabilitate, or palliate to maintain the physiologic and psychosocial stability of patients across the life span.
- Perform vigilant assessment and monitoring of the patient's condition to prevent failure to rescue.

- Synthesize and prioritize information in order to take immediate and decisive evidence-based, patient-focused action using clinical judgment and clinical inquiry.
- Anticipate and respond with confidence, and adapt to rapidly changing patient conditions.
- Respond to the unique and diverse needs of patients and families coping with unanticipated illness or injury and treatment.
- Advocate for patient and family choices in quality-of-life and end-of-life decisions.
- Prepare for safe transitions of care while promoting health and health equity and addressing social determinants of health
- Establish and maintain a healthy work environment that is safe, respectful, healing, and caring for nurses, peers, patients, families, and the interprofessional team.
- Promote and maintain care for self and coworkers to prevent burnout, compassion fatigue and moral distress, and to promote nurse well-being.[6]
- Promote the financial contribution of progressive care nursing through appropriate resource utilization, financial stewardship, innovation, and efficiency.
- Incorporate tools, such as early warning systems, artificial intelligence, and surveillance systems, to improve patient safety and reduce nurses' workload.[7]
- Demonstrate the value of progressive care nursing and its contribution to quality outcomes, patient safety, and the financial health of the organization.

It is essential that nurses and all other members of the team caring for patients be vigilant and alert to monitor and respond appropriately to changes in patients' health or illness.

Practice Population

Progressive care nurses provide care for patients based on their unique needs across the continuum of care. These patients have acute and/or chronic complex needs, their patients' unique comorbidities, and are at high risk for instability.

ACUTELY AND/OR CHRONICALLY ILL OR INJURED PATIENTS

Progressive care nurses practice in settings where patients require complex assessment and therapies, moderately high-intensity interventions, and high-level nursing vigilance. Patient characteristics in this population can be defined along the health vulnerability to illness and injury continuum described by the AACN Synergy Model, as follows:[5]

The Synergy Model was originally developed for the critical care patient. The Progressive Care Scope and Standards Task Force has adapted Synergy Model Nurse level 3 characteristics[5] as generally applying to patients needing progressive care. Sub bullets provide examples of these patients and the needs for each characteristic.

- Resilience – the capacity to return to a restorative level of functioning using compensatory coping mechanisms; the ability to recover quickly after an insult or injury

  Example:

  Patients have a moderate ability to initiate some degree of compensation and have moderate reserves.

- Vulnerability – susceptibility to actual or potential stressors that may adversely affect patient outcome

  Examples:

  1. Patients range between somewhat susceptible and somewhat protected to actual or potential stresses.
  2. The patient needs trust and rapport with the nurse and their interactions to help overcome vulnerability and develop resilience.

- Stability – the ability to maintain steady-state equilibrium

  Examples:

  1. Patients are able to maintain a steady state for a limited period of time and have some responsiveness to therapies.
  2. These patients have a risk of instability.

- Complexity – the intricate entanglement of 2 or more systems (eg, body, mind, cultural, family, therapies)

  Example:

  Patients have moderately involved complexity dynamics that could include comorbidities, social determinants of health, health literacy, and developmental age/stage. Family dynamics are also considered moderately involved.

- Resource availability – the body of resources (eg, technical, fiscal, personal, psychological, social) that the patient, family, and community bring to the situation

  Examples:

  1. Patients and their families may have moderate resources but need assistance with knowledge and skills, financial support, personal and psychological support services, and social system resources.
  2. The patient's perspective will depend on their access to health equity and how social determinants of health affect them.

- Participation in care – extent to which the patient and family engage in aspects of decision making

  Example:

  Patients and their families have a moderate level of participation and need assistance for care.

- Participation in decision-making processes – extent to which the patient and family engage in decision making, including patient choices and preferences

    Example:

    Patients and their families have a moderate level of participation in shared decision making and will seek input and advice from others in shared decision making.

- Predictability – a summative characteristic that allows one to expect a certain course of events or illness

    Example:

    Patients are moderately predictable in their response to health care interventions.

THE PRACTICE ENVIRONMENT

Progressive care nurses practice in settings where patients require complex assessments and interventions. These settings are not defined by the needs of the patient or the patient's location in a designated unit. These patients may be in settings where the boundaries of specialty practice are often fluid, due to their changing needs. Based on *AACN Certification Corporation Practice Analysis of Progressive Nursing Care*[3] and the expert opinion of the Progressive Care Scope and Standards Task Force, typical areas considered to be progressive care but may not be labeled as such include telemetry, stepdown, intermediate, emergency department, long-term acute care, and procedural areas. Nurses lead and participate in collaborative interprofessional teams to create safe, respectful, healing, and caring environments in which:

- Patients and families' values and preferences are central to the development of informed care decisions made in collaboration with and using the expertise of the interprofessional health care team.
- Ethical decision making is supported, fostered, and promoted.
- Nurses are valued and committed partners on the interprofessional team in decision making that impacts patient care, the practice environment, and organizational operations.
- Nurses act as advocates on behalf of patients, families, and communities.
- Collaboration and collegiality are embraced.
- Practice is based on research and best evidence.
- Nursing clinical judgment helps evaluate system information that influences patient care such as clinical decision support tools and early warning systems that use artificial intelligence.
- Leadership skill development is fostered at all levels.

- Professional and organizational leadership encourages and supports effective decision making, lifelong learning, and professional growth.
- Individual talents and resources are optimized.
- Innovation, creativity, and clinical inquiry are recognized and valued.
- Principles of equity, diversity and inclusion are recognized, supported, and respected.
- Skilled communication is demonstrated at all levels.
- A professional practice model drives delivery of nursing care.
- Burnout is recognized; self-care and caregiver wellness are prioritized and supported.
- Nurses are recognized and recognize others for the value each brings to the work of the organization.
- The standards of a healthy work environment[8] are implemented to support the health and safety of the interprofessional team.
- Zero tolerance for inappropriate behavior, incivility, discrimination, bullying, verbal abuse, or violent behavior is the expectation and supported by organizational policy.
- Efforts to reduce and eliminate implicit or unconscious bias are supported and guided by best practices.
- Appropriate nurse staffing ensures the match of patient needs and nurse competencies to promote safety and quality outcomes.[9]

Such healthy work environments foster recognition and advance the authority, autonomy, and accountability of progressive care nurses to achieve equitable, optimal outcomes.

RESPECT, EQUITY, DIVERSITY, INCLUSION, AND SOCIAL JUSTICE

Respect for oneself and others is essential to nurses implementing the practice of caring using the principles of equity, diversity, inclusion, and social justice.[2] When respect is present it allows nurses to learn about others cultures and practice cultural humility. Social justice is also critically important for nurses to learn about and commit to, in order to advocate and address social determinants of health and promote well-being in all settings.[2] Progressive care nurses must commit to learning that strengthens their own understanding of these concepts and how best to advocate on behalf of patients and families to promote equity, diversity, and inclusion. For more information on these concepts, please see ANA's *Nursing: Scope and Standards of Practice*, 4th edition.[2]

EDUCATION AND PROFESSIONAL COMPETENCE

The public expects nursing competence. Professional competence demonstrated throughout one's nursing career requires a commitment to the process of lifelong learning, personal reviews of practice, inviting peer reviews, and undergoing performance evaluations.[2] The competencies of progressive care nurses build on the foundation of their basic nursing education and require additional knowledge, skills, and expertise beyond what is learned in general nursing practice and educational programs. The competencies required by nurses caring for patients are defined in the AACN Synergy Model.[4] These requisite competencies are Clinical Judgment, Advocacy and Moral Agency, Caring Practices, Collaboration, Systems Thinking, Response to Diversity, Facilitation of Learning, and Clinical Inquiry. Nurses' competencies are derived from patients' needs. These needs take into account a patient's physical, social, psychological, cultural, and spiritual realms. The Synergy Model's nurse competencies helped develop *AACN Competence Framework for Progressive and Critical Care Nursing Practice: Initial Competency 2022*.[10] This framework establishes the national standard for entry-level competence of a progressive care nurse.

Orientation and education that validate the competence of the nurse are needed to provide safe, quality care. Two tools to support validation are available for progressive care nursing practice: *AACN Competence Framework and Toolkit* for the overall assessment of initial competence and the AACN Knowledge Assessment Tool for Progressive Care[11] to assess entry-level knowledge competence. Ensuring progressive care nurse competence includes support for precepting, mentoring, and nurse progression along the novice to expert continuum. Length of orientation, training/cross-training, and/or residency and content should be tailored to the specific patients cared for on the unit and the individual nurse's needs, education, and experience. Education, orientation, and training should focus on development of the nurse's competence in caring for the population of patients served.

Nursing care reflects an integration of KSAs, experience, and attitudes to meet the needs of patients and their families. The Institute of Medicine (now called National Academy of Medicine), in its report titled *The Future of Nursing: Leading Change, Advancing Health*, recommended that the proportion of nurses with a baccalaureate degree be increased to 80% by the year 2020.[12] *The Future of Nursing 2020-2030: Charting a Path to Achieve Health Equity*, Chapter 7: Educating Nurses for the Future reaffirms the goal of 80% baccalaureate-prepared nurses. As the proportion of BSN-prepared nurses increases in the nurse-to-patient numbers, evidence shows improvements in health outcomes.[13] Advancement to the level of baccalaureate education should be the goal for nurses currently entering practice and for those with associate-level or diploma education. Employers and educational institutions should support the ability to achieve educational advancement.[13]

Self-Determination and Professional Identity

According to ANA, "the development of professional competence enhances the concept of self-determination and helps promote formation and demonstration of professional identity."[2] Commitment to lifelong learning and professional development can be demonstrated by the attainment of continuing education, participation in professional opportunities, and achieving higher academic degrees, advanced education, and/or specialty certifications and credentials. This achievement exemplifies the nurse's commitment to self-determination, the development of professional identity and professional career development, and dedication to safe, quality, and equitable patient care in this constantly changing environment.[14] A nurse's concept of self-determination continues to develop throughout their career based on their exposure to the profession, their focus on caring, and the components of the regulation of their practice.[2]

REGULATION

There are 5 key components of regulation of professional nursing practice, according to ANA's *Nursing Scope and Standards of Practice*, 4th edition. (2021).[2] These key components are evidence, nursing practice, influencers, quality, and safety. The key influencers that regulate progressive care nursing practice include scope and standards of practice and professional performance, a code of ethics, specialty certification, nurse practice acts with rules and regulations, and institutional policies and procedures.

Nursing Scope of Practice, Standards of Practice, and Specialty Certification

Scope and standards of practice are set by professional nursing organizations. ANA's *Nursing: Scope and Standards of Practice*[2] and this document provide the foundation for specialty organizations to define practice within the specialty and patient population. Certification of progressive care nurses is a formal recognition of knowledge, skills, and experience based on national standards and validated by a practice analysis. AACN recommends that nurses be certified in their specialty. Certification and certification renewal provide validation to consumers, employers, patients and families, and nurses themselves that they have demonstrated achievement of standards identified by a nursing specialty to promote optimal health outcomes.[14]

Nurse Practice Acts and Rules and Regulations

The practice of progressive care nurses is regulated externally. Nurse practice acts are administered under the authority of state governments to ensure public safety. The progressive care nurse is licensed as an RN in the state in which the nurse practices and is subject to that state's legal constraints and regulations. The only exemptions exist in the Department of Veterans Affairs, the Department of Defense, and the Indian Health Service. Currently, nurses working virtually are subject to regulations in the state where the patient is located.[15]

Institutional Policies, Procedures, and Guidelines

The nurse is also regulated by institutional policies, procedures, and guidelines that define practice. While nurses may be educated to perform specific skills, it is essential for them to know the privileging actions and/or restrictions imposed by the policies, procedures, and guidelines of their facility.

ETHICAL PRACTICE

Progressive care nurses engage in ethical practice and base their decisions and actions on their commitment to patients and families, consistent with ANA's *Code of Ethics for Nurses with Interpretive Statements*[16] and AACN's core values.[17] Progressive care nurses practice according to the AACN core values of integrity, inclusion, transformation, leadership, and relationships. Their practice also acknowledges dignity, autonomy, diversity, cultural beliefs, privacy, and confidentiality, including the health information and health literacy of patients and families. Culturally safe and competent care requires a continual appraisal of one's personal and professional values and how they may impact issue interpretation and decision making.[2] Nurses need to be aware of indications of burnout, compassion fatigue, and/or moral distress/injury in themselves and in others. Nurses are equally obligated to advocate for and maintain the health, safety, and well-being of themselves and others. This obligation must be supported by the organization and necessitates the pursuit and development of healthy work environments.[9]

In addition, progressive care nurses advocate for and collaborate with the patient, family, and interprofessional team in care decisions. This collaboration includes information sharing with the patient and family regarding the options of palliative and end-of-life care supporting the goal of patient- and family-centered care. The obligation of advocacy continues into the realm of research, whether in the conduct of, participation in, or facilitation of research and scholarly inquiry.

Nurses caring for patients also have an ethical obligation to maintain patient safety by reporting and, if necessary, intervening to protect patients from any unsafe conduct by members of the interprofessional team. This obligation applies not only to specific actions, but also to the overall maintenance of professional competence and personal health. When an unhealthy work environment is evident, the nurse must work collaboratively with their organization to seek to determine the cause and facilitate a resolution. Actions such as violence and incivility among peers or poor communication and collaboration among members of the interprofessional team must be addressed collaboratively to ensure a healthy work environment and the safety of the patient. Zero tolerance for violence by team members and/or patients and families is required and must be supported by the organization.

CONCLUSION

This scope of practice document clarifies the practice role of progressive care nurses when caring for patients and families and the impact of the work environment on the provision of nursing care. Progressive care nurses face unique challenges for patients with complex needs, who may present at any point across the life span with multiple comorbidities and who may face end-of-life care decisions. Care of these patients and families requires increased vigilance in a health care system with rapidly changing technology and often limited resources. Transitions of care across the continuum require collaboration and communication within the interprofessional team. Progressive care nurses must maintain competence in all of these dimensions to achieve optimal patient outcomes.

REFERENCES

1. Curley MAQ. *Synergy: The Unique Relationship Between Nurses and Patients.* Sigma Theta Tau International; 2007.

2. American Nurses Association. *Nursing: Scope and Standards of Practice.* 4th ed. American Nurses Association; 2021. Accessed May 15, 2024. https://www.nursingworld.org/nurses-books/nursing-scope-and-standards-of-practice-4th-edit/

3. AACN Certification Corporation. 2023 Practice analysis of the progressive care nurse.

4. American Association of Critical-Care Nurses. AACN Synergy Model for Patient Care. Accessed May 29, 2024. https://www.aacn.org/~/media/aacn-website/nursing-excellence/standards/aacnsynergymodelforpatientcare.pdf?la=en

5. Johnson BH. Promoting patient- and family-centered care through personal stories. *Acad Med.* 2016:91(3):297–300. Accessed May 28, 2024. doi:10.1097/ACM.0000000000001086

6. Partners for Nurse Staffing Think Tank. Stress injury continuum. https://www.nursingworld.org/practice-policy/nurse-staffing/nurse-staffing-task-force/nurse-staffing-think-tank/

7. Partners for Nurse Staffing Think Tank. Priority topics and recommendations. https://www.nursingworld.org/practice-policy/nurse-staffing/nurse-staffing-task-force/nurse-staffing-think-tank/

8. Barden C, ed. *AACN Standards for Establishing and Sustaining Healthy Work Environments: A Journey to Excellence.* 2nd ed. American Association of Critical-Care Nurses; 2016. https://www.aacn.org/nursing-excellence/standards/aacn-standards-for-establishing-and-sustaining-healthy-work-environments

9. Delgado SA, Good V, Barden C, Cassidy L, eds. *AACN Standards for Appropriate Staffing in Adult Critical Care.* American Association of Critical-Care Nurses; 2024. Accessed June 10, 2024. https://www.aacn.org/~/media/aacn-website/nursing-excellence/standards/aacn-standards-for-appropriate-staffing-in-adult-critical-care.pdf

10. American Association of Critical-Care Nurses. *AACN Competence Framework for Progressive and Critical Care: Initial Competency 2022.* Accessed May 14, 2024. https://www.aacn.org/nursing-excellence/standards/aacn-competence-framework-for-progressive-and-critical-care

11. American Association of Critical-Care Nurses. AACN Knowledge Assessment Tool. Accessed June 10, 2024. https://www.aacn.org/education/knowledge-assessment-tool?tab=Single-Site%20LearnCenter

12. Institute of Medicine. *The Future of Nursing: Leading Change, Advancing Health.* National Academies Press; 2010. Accessed June 10, 2024. https://nap.nationalacademies.org/read/12956/chapter/1#xv

13. National Academies of Sciences, Engineering, and Medicine. *The Future of Nursing 2020-2030: Charting a Path to Achieve Health Equity.* National Academies Press; 2021. Accessed June 10, 2024. https://doi.org/10.17226/25982

14. AACN Certification Corporation. Value of certification. Accessed June 10, 2024. http://www.aacn.org/wd/certifications/content/benefitstoptempnrs.pcms?menu=certification

15. National Council of State Boards of Nursing. Nurse licensure compact. Accessed June 10, 2024. https://www.ncsbn.org/nurse-licensure-compact.htm

16. American Nurses Association. *Code of Ethics for Nurses with Interpretive Statements.* Nursesbooks.org; 2015.

17. American Association of Critical-Care Nurses. AACN core values. Accessed June 10, 2024. https://www.aacn.org/about-aacn

STANDARDS OF PRACTICE FOR PROGRESSIVE CARE NURSING

INTRODUCTION

The standards of practice and accompanying standards of professional performance are intended to support the *Scope of Practice for Progressive Care Nurses.* These standards apply to the care that progressive care nurses provide for all patients. The competencies describe how each standard is met. Nurses practice with these competencies based on their level of experience and professional development.

STANDARDS OF PRACTICE

The standards of practice for progressive care nurses also build on ANA's *Nursing: Scope and Standards of Practice*[1] to delineate expectations in this specialty environment. Progressive care nurses are expected to practice in accordance with the competencies identified in both documents. The professional practice of progressive care nurses is characterized by the application of relevant theories, research, and evidence-based guidelines to diagnose and treat human responses to injury and illness. The nursing process is used as the framework; it includes assessment, diagnosis, outcomes identification, planning, implementation, and evaluation.

The professional practice of progressive care nurses is characterized by the application of relevant theories, research, and evidence-based guidelines.

STANDARD 1

ASSESSMENT

The nurse obtains comprehensive data and information pertinent to the situation and/or patient's health.

COMPETENCIES

- Collects data and information from the patient, family, other health care providers, and the community, as appropriate, to develop a holistic picture of the patient's needs or condition
- Prioritizes data and information collection based on the patient's characteristics related to the immediate condition and anticipated needs related to the acuity of the patient
- Uses valid evidence-based assessment techniques, instruments, and tools based on the need for vigilance to identify patterns and variances in the stability of the patient's condition
- Completes an initial assessment and reassesses based on the patient's condition due to their high risk for instability
- Conducts a learning assessment to assess health literacy and social determinants of health
- Documents data and information in a clear and retrievable format

STANDARD 2 | DIAGNOSIS

The nurse analyzes and synthesizes information and data from the assessment in determining actual or potential diagnoses, conditions, problems, and issues relevant to care.

COMPETENCIES

- Validates diagnoses, conditions, problems, and other issues with the patient, family, and other health care providers
- Documents diagnoses, conditions, problems, and other issues in a clear and retrievable format

STANDARD 3 | OUTCOMES IDENTIFICATION

The nurse using their clinical expertise identifies outcomes in collaboration with the patient, family, and interprofessional team.

COMPETENCIES

- Identifies preferences and values in formulating patient- and family-centered outcomes that meet diversity and cultural needs in collaboration with the patient, family, and interprofessional team
- Considers associated risks, benefits, best available evidence, social determinants of health, and essential costs when formulating outcomes to avoid placing unnecessary burdens on the patient and/or family
- Documents identified outcomes as measurable goals in a clear and retrievable format

STANDARD 4

PLANNING

The nurse uses their clinical expertise and develops a collaborative plan that identifies strategies and alternatives to attain outcomes.

COMPETENCIES

- Uses clinical judgment and inquiry to develop an individualized plan
- Collaborates with the patient, family, and interprofessional team to develop the plan
- Establishes priorities and continuity of care including transfer of information and handoffs per the plan
- Includes strategies for health equity, health promotion and education, and prevention of complications or injury
- Considers associated risks, benefits, best evidence, resources, and cost when developing the plan
- Plans for transitions of care regarding escalation or de-escalation of care
- Documents and provides handoff of the plan in a clear and retrievable manner

Standards 2, 3, and 4 address the competencies needed to determine diagnoses, identify outcomes, and develop a collaborative plan.

STANDARD

5

IMPLEMENTATION

The nurse implements the plan in coordination with the patient, family, and interprofessional team. Implementation also includes nurse-coordinated care delivery and employing strategies to teach and promote health and wellness.

COMPETENCIES

- Employs strategies to promote and maintain a safe environment, including a healthy work environment
- Uses clinical judgment to implement the nursing process to enhance acute care outcomes in progressive care nursing practice
- Intervenes to prevent and minimize complications and alleviate suffering
- Facilitates learning for patients, families, and the community using appropriate methods based on needs and health literacy
- Provides age- and developmentally appropriate care with respect to diversity
- Uses approaches that are inclusive, equitable, and culturally and psychologically safe
- Prepares the patient and family for transitions of care regarding escalation or de-escalation of care
- Documents implementation in a clear and retrievable format

STANDARD

6

EVALUATION

The nurse evaluates progress toward attainment of outcomes.

COMPETENCIES

- Conducts systematic and ongoing evaluations using evidence-based techniques, tools, and instruments
- Evaluates patient and family understanding of education and transition of care planning using evidence-based assessments
- Collaborates with the patient, family, and interprofessional team in the evaluation process
- Revises the assessment, diagnoses, outcomes identification, plan, and interventions based on information gained during the evaluation process
- Documents the results of evaluations in a clear and retrievable format

REFERENCE

American Nurses Association. *Nursing: Scope and Standards of Practice.* 4th ed. American Nurses Association; 2021.

EXAMPLES OF APPLYING THE STANDARDS OF PRACTICE FOR PROGRESSIVE CARE NURSING

These vignettes provide examples of how the 6 Standards of Practice competencies are demonstrated in progressive care nursing practice.

STANDARDS 1 AND 2 – ASSESSMENT AND DIAGNOSIS COMPETENCIES ARE DEMONSTRATED IN THE FOLLOWING 2 VIGNETTES.

Standard of Practice 1: Assessment - The nurse obtains comprehensive data and information pertinent to the situation and/or patient's health.

COMPETENCIES

- Collects data and information from the patient, family, other health care providers, and the community, as appropriate, to develop a holistic picture of the patient's needs or conditions
- Prioritizes data and information collection based on patient characteristics related to the immediate condition and anticipated needs related to the acuity of the patient
- Uses valid evidence-based assessment techniques, instruments, and tools based on the need for vigilance to identify patterns and variances in the stability of the patient's condition
- Completes an initial assessment and reassesses based on the patient's condition due to the high risk for instability

Standard of Practice 2: Diagnosis - The nurse analyzes and synthesizes information and data from the assessment in determining actual or potential diagnoses, conditions, problems, and other issues relevant to care.

COMPETENCIES

- Validates diagnoses, conditions, problems, and other issues with the patient, family, and other health care providers

ASSESSMENT AND DIAGNOSIS, VIGNETTE #1

The progressive care unit (PCU) nurse receives report on a patient who is transferring from the intensive care unit (ICU). The ICU nurse states that the patient was admitted for hypoxemic respiratory failure due to heart failure exacerbation, which resulted in the patient requiring mechanical ventilation for 3 days and continuous infusion of a diuretic. The patient was extubated yesterday and has been maintaining oxygen saturations greater than 92% on 4 L of oxygen via nasal cannula (NC).

The patient arrives in the PCU, and the nurse conducts a full physical assessment. The nurse auscultates faint rhonchi in the posterior bilateral lower lobes. The patient's pulse oximetry reading is 95% on 4 L NC oxygen.

Two hours after arrival at the PCU, the patient's cardiac monitor alarms for oxygen desaturation to 85%. The nurse enters the room and assesses that the patient is dyspneic. The nurse increases the oxygen to 6 L NC and auscultates the patient's lungs, which now have diffuse rhonchi. The patient's deep breathing during auscultation elicits a strong cough that produces a large amount of thick yellow sputum. Based on these findings, the nurse suspects that the patient has developed alterations in respiration due to ventilator-associated pneumonia and notifies the provider. A chest x-ray is ordered that shows pulmonary infiltrates consistent with pneumonia, and the provider orders the patient to be started on IV antibiotics.

ASSESSMENT AND DIAGNOSIS, VIGNETTE #2

A progressive care registered nurse (RN) working on a cardiac surgical stepdown unit was caring for an older adult patient after their aortic valve replacement surgery. The patient was 2 days post-surgery and had been transferred from the cardiac surgery intensive care unit (CSICU) earlier in the nurse's shift. The patient's postoperative time in the CSICU was uneventful except for a brief period of atrial fibrillation, during which the patient was treated with an intravenous infusion of amiodarone, which successfully converted the patient's irregular rhythm back to sinus rhythm. The patient was transferred from the CSICU to cardiac surgical stepdown and connected to a temporary pacemaker via ventricle epicardial wires at a rate of 40, mA of 5, and sensitivity of 1.2. The patient had not required any pacing via the epicardial temporary pacemaker since the patient arrived on the stepdown unit.

The patient was ambulating in the hallway with the progressive care RN and patient care associate (PCA) when the patient reported feeling suddenly dizzy and lightheaded. The RN and PCA assisted the patient to a chair in the hallway and took the patient's vital signs. The patient had marked hypotension of 82/54 and was determined to be in atrial fibrillation with a rapid ventricular response of 136 beats/minute. The RN and PCA quickly called for help and assisted the patient back to their room in a wheelchair.

Upon returning the patient to bed, the RN noticed there was also a significant increase in the patient's chest tube output, with frank red blood now appearing in the drainage chambers. The RN was quickly concerned about the patient's compensatory presentation with hypotension, rapid atrial fibrillation paired with increased chest tube output, and report of dizziness. The RN auscultated the patient's lungs and found them clear; however, when the RN auscultated the patient's heart sounds, the RN heard muffled heart sounds. The RN also noticed the patient's jugular veins were distended, and the patient was sweating with new shortness of breath.

The cardiac surgery advanced practice nurse (APN) was urgently called to the bedside. The RN reported the patient's events, vital signs, and assessment to the cardiac surgery APN and verbalized concern for possible cardiac tamponade. The APN acknowledged the RN's concerns and assessment and ordered an infusion of albumin, stat labs, and a bedside echocardiogram and called the on-call cardiac surgeon. The bedside echocardiogram revealed a large pericardial effusion with tamponade, and the patient was urgently brought to the operating room by the progressive care RN and cardiac surgery APN for an emergent pericardiocentesis.

STANDARDS 3 AND 4 – OUTCOMES IDENTIFICATION AND PLANNING COMPETENCIES ARE DEMONSTRATED IN THE FOLLOWING VIGNETTE.

Standard 3: Outcomes Identification - The nurse using their clinical expertise identifies outcomes in collaboration with the patient, family, and interprofessional team.

COMPETENCIES

- Identifies preferences and values in formulating patient- and family-centered outcomes that meet diversity and cultural needs in collaboration with the patient, family, and interprofessional team
- Considers associated risks, benefits, best available evidence, social determinants of health, and essential costs when formulating outcomes to avoid placing unnecessary burdens on the patient and/or family
- Documents identified outcomes as measurable goals in a clear and retrievable format

Standard 4: Planning - The nurse uses their clinical expertise and develops a collaborative plan that identifies strategies and alternatives to attain outcomes.

COMPETENCIES

- Uses clinical judgment and inquiry to develop an individualized plan
- Collaborates with the patient, family, and interprofessional team to develop the plan
- Establishes priorities and continuity of care, including transfer of information and handoffs per the plan
- Includes strategies for health equity, health promotion and education, and prevention of complications or injury
- Considers associated risks, benefits, best evidence, resources, and cost when developing the plan

OUTCOMES IDENTIFICATION AND PLANNING, VIGNETTE #3

A novice nurse in the progressive care unit (PCU) is expressing frustration to a more experienced colleague/former preceptor about how they're seeing more patients readmitted to the hospital due to what they perceive as a lack of adherence to the medication regimen. Specifically, the patient with diabetes who has a Russian language preference is back again for high blood glucose level.

The experienced nurse empathizes with the novice nurse's frustration and suggests why some patients are unable to adhere to their diabetic medications. They explore possible options, including misconceptions about side effects, financial constraints, lack of insurance coverage, limited access to pharmacies or prescription mail programs, competing priorities, language barriers, and health literacy challenges. This discussion of the impact of social determinants of health prompts the novice nurse to express a desire to do a better job exploring how to help patients identify and overcome these potential barriers while they are in the hospital.

Together, the 2 nurses identified the desired outcome of improved medication understanding and adherence for frequently readmitted patients, and they collaborated to establish specific goals for interacting with this patient and others:

- Initiate open and nonjudgmental conversations with patients about their medication experiences, exploring potential barriers to adherence.
- Collaborate with the interdisciplinary team to facilitate access to resources that will help address or mitigate barriers.
- Foster the patient's engagement and self-advocacy in medication management to promote long-term adherence and improved health outcomes.
- Document the patient's concerns accurately to inform the rest of the team of the patient's status.

Later in the shift, the novice nurse initiates a discussion using a Russian-speaking interpreter and discovers how challenging it has been for the patient to pay for insulin on top of covering their family's expenses. The patient worried about getting access to the pills and insulin that they need when they go home while also ensuring the bills are paid. The nurse takes the opportunity to ensure there is a social work and case management consultation ordered for the patient. The nurse encourages the patient to share these concerns with the medical team during rounds and documents a nursing note to ensure the rest of the team is informed. The nurse continues to approach future patients with these goals in mind.

REFERENCE

National Academies of Sciences, Engineering, and Medicine. *The Future of Nursing 2020-2030: Charting a Path to Achieve Health Equity*. National Academies Press; 2021. https://nap.nationalacademies.org/read/25982/chapter/1#:~:text=Suggested%20Citation%3A%22Front%20Matter.,DC%3A%20The%20National%20Academies%20Press

STANDARDS 4, 5 AND 6 – PLANNING, IMPLEMENTATION, AND EVALUATION COMPETENCIES ARE DEMONSTRATED IN THE FOLLOWING VIGNETTE.

Standard 4: Planning

The nurse uses their clinical expertise and develops a collaborative plan that identifies strategies and alternatives to attain outcomes.

COMPETENCIES

- Uses clinical judgment and inquiry to develop an individualized plan
- Collaborates with the patient, family, and interprofessional team to develop the plan
- Establishes priorities and continuity of care, including transfer of information and handoffs per the plan
- Includes strategies for health equity, health promotion and education, and prevention of complications or injury
- Plans for transitions of care regarding escalation or de-escalation of care

EXAMPLES

Standard 5: Implementation

The nurse implements the plan in coordination with the patient, family, and interprofessional team. Implementation also includes nurse-coordinated care delivery and employing strategies to teach and promote health and wellness.

COMPETENCIES

- Intervenes to prevent and minimize complications and alleviate suffering
- Facilitates learning for patients, families, and the community using appropriate methods based on needs and health literacy
- Provides age- and developmentally appropriate care with respect to diversity
- Uses approaches that are inclusive, equitable, and culturally and psychologically safe
- Prepares the patient and family for transitions of care regarding escalation or de-escalation of care
- Documents implementation in a clear and retrievable format

Standard 6: Evaluation

The nurse evaluates progress toward attainment of outcomes.

COMPETENCIES

- Evaluates patient and family understanding of education and transition of care planning using evidence-based assessments
- Collaborates with the patient, family, and interprofessional team in the evaluation process

PLANNING, IMPLEMENTATION, AND EVALUATION, VIGNETTE #4

A patient with a Spanish-language preference underwent coronary artery bypass graft surgery times 4 vessels and was deemed ready for discharge by the cardiac surgery team. The progressive care nurse planned to have an interpreter present for discharge teaching, since they knew the patient's preferred language was Spanish. The nurse asked an in-person Spanish interpreter to help review discharge instructions with the patient and their significant other, which included weight restrictions, diet, medications, incision care, and upcoming appointments. The nurse also ensured that the printed discharge instructions were in Spanish and at a reading level that matched the patient's health literacy level. Since the patient also had diabetes, the nurse emphasized maintaining glucose control to help the incisions heal properly. After reviewing the discharge instructions, the nurse asked the patient and their significant other to teach back their discharge instructions to ensure that they understood the information and knew when to call the cardiac surgery office for questions or go to the nearest emergency department for emergencies, such as chest pain.

A patient with a Spanish-language preference underwent coronary artery bypass graft surgery and was deemed ready for discharge. What was the progressive care nurse's next step?

STANDARDS OF PROFESSIONAL PERFORMANCE FOR PROGRESSIVE CARE NURSING

INTRODUCTION

Standards of professional performance describe competencies related to ethics, advocacy, respectful and equitable practice, communication, collaboration, leadership, education, scholarly inquiry, quality of practice, professional practice evaluation, resource stewardship, and environmental health.

The competency statements, which describe how the standards are met, are not in order according to level of importance. Nurses practice with these competencies based on their level of experience and professional development.

These standards are meant to be used in conjunction with *AACN Scope and Standards of Practice for Progressive Care Nursing Practice* and ANA's *Nursing: Scope and Standards of Practice*[1] and do not stand alone in describing the practice of progressive care nurses. They are expected to practice in accordance with the competencies identified in both documents.

STANDARD

7

ETHICS

The nurse integrates ethics into all aspects of practice.

COMPETENCIES

Ethical accountability for patients

- Practices as guided by ANA's *Code of Ethics for Nurses with Interpretive Statements*[2] and AACN's core values[3]
- Promotes ethical accountability and integrity in relationships, patient confidentiality and privacy, organizational decisions, and stewardship of resources in consideration of the dynamic nature of care transitions and patient acuity
- Advocates for the concerns of the patient, family, and community
- Supports the patient and family in self-determination and informed decision making
- Maintains respect for patient autonomy, dignity, values, beliefs, and rights at all times
- Delivers care in an inclusive, equitable, culturally, and psychologically safe manner that meets the diverse needs of the patient, family, and community
- Uses available resources in making ethical decisions
- Reports unethical, illegal, incompetent, or impaired practices
- Maintains a therapeutic and professional nurse/patient relationship within appropriate role boundaries
- Contributes to resolving ethical issues involving the patient, family, and interprofessional team
- Questions health care practice when necessary for safety and quality improvement
- Uses patient information and data in an ethically responsible manner
- Collaborates with the interprofessional team to promote transitions of care, palliative care, and end-of-life discussions, decisions, and care

STANDARD

7 ETHICS (CONT'D)

The nurse integrates ethics into all aspects of practice.

COMPETENCIES (CONT'D)

Ethical Obligations to Self

- Demonstrates a commitment to self-care and self-advocacy
- Recognizes moral distress, burnout, and/or compassion fatigue in self and others
- Seeks appropriate support and resources to address moral distress, burnout, and compassion fatigue
- Fosters holistic well-being in self and others[4]
- Identifies personal beliefs and values, biases, and cultural values that may affect ethical obligations to patients
- Seeks appropriate resources and support to address personal beliefs and values, biases, and cultural values that may affect ethical obligations to patients
- Promotes development and sustainment of a healthy work environment
- Shows zero tolerance for workplace violence,[5] including bullying, verbal abuse, discrimination, and incivility[6]
- Promotes a just culture and supports colleagues as second victims when errors in patient care occur

STANDARD

8 ADVOCACY

The nurse demonstrates advocacy in all roles and settings.

COMPETENCIES

- Promotes patient preferences while preserving the patients' dignity and rights while involving them in the shared decision-making process
- Holds organizations/individuals accountable for workplace violence/incivility
- Advocates for equitable and appropriate resources that enhance and support nursing practice, patient safety, and quality of care
- Champions the allocation of resources specific to the patient's needs to support outcomes beyond hospitalization
- Reinforces evidence-based practice as the basis for progressive care nursing
- Leverages progressive care nurse expertise to promote equitable health care delivery and mitigate barriers to equitable health care delivery
- Serves as a voice for vulnerable populations, advocating for policies and interventions that promote health equity
- Advocates for nurse behavioral and mental health support and suicide prevention
- Promotes regulatory and health policy that impacts health care and progressive care nursing practice
- Encourages progressive care nurses involvement in professional organizations' advocacy efforts, community initiatives, legislative health policy, regulatory policies, or advocacy campaigns that affect progressive care practice
- Supports making data more complete, higher quality, more accessible, and more representative of all people to promote health data equity
- Advocates for escalation of care based on the needs of the patient

STANDARD 9

RESPECTFUL AND EQUITABLE PRACTICE

The nurse practices with cultural humility and inclusiveness.

COMPETENCIES

- Identifies opportunities for lifelong learning to understand values, beliefs, heritage, cultural preferences, worldviews, choices, unconscious biases, and decision-making processes of self, peers, and population served
- Identifies skills and tools needed for the specific culture, literacy, and language of the progressive care population served

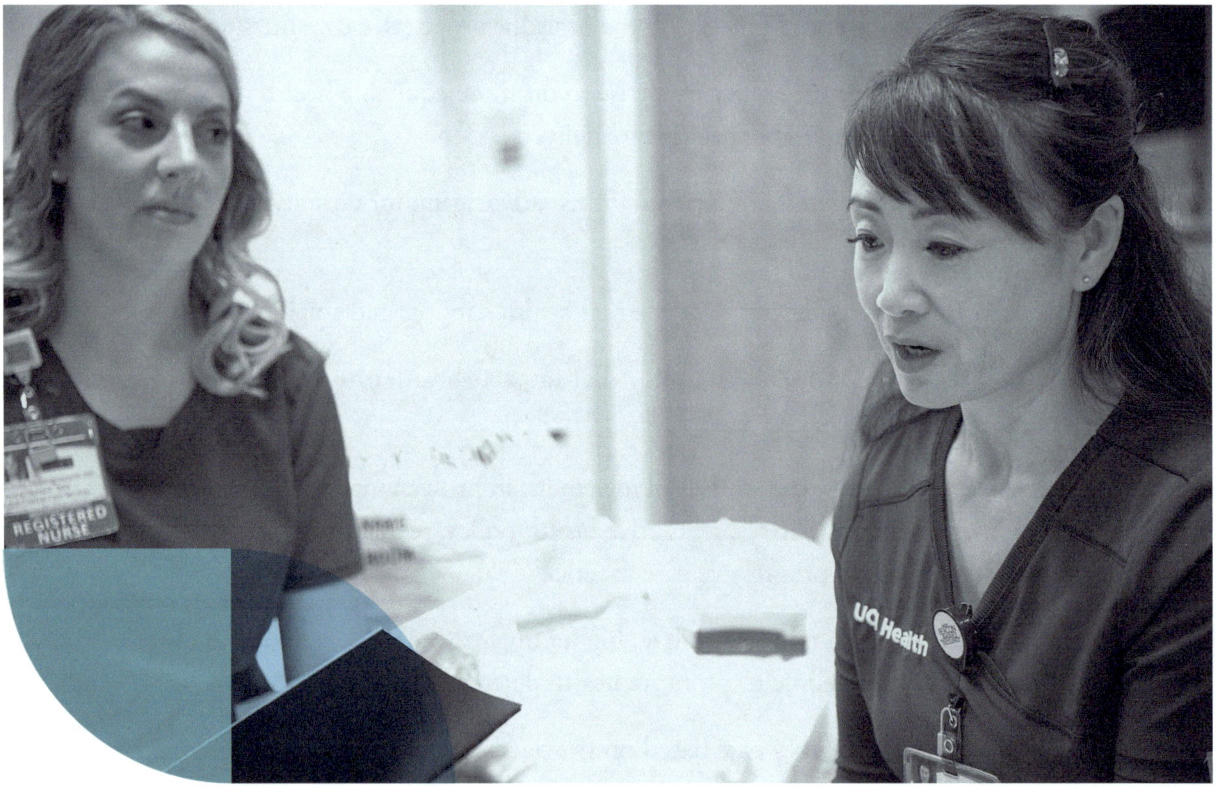

STANDARD 10 COMMUNICATION

The nurse communicates effectively in all areas of practice.

COMPETENCIES

- Reflects on personal communication style
- Solicits feedback to continually improve communication and conflict-resolution skills
- Implements feedback in practice
- Assesses communication preferences and abilities of patients, families, and the interprofessional team
- Practices interprofessional skilled communication appropriate to the situation and platform
- Minimizes risks associated with patient handoffs, transfers, and transitions of care
- Uses validated language access, communication, transitions of care, and handoff tool resources when appropriate[7]
- Assesses health literacy and learning style, and language preferences for patients and families
- Conveys accurate information to patients, families, and the interprofessional team in a way they can understand
- Confirms communication is heard and the message is understood
- Validates own understanding of the rationale for care processes and decisions
- Clarifies the rationale for care processes and decisions with others, as appropriate
- Contributes professional nursing perspective in discussions with the interprofessional team
- Follows the chain of command to report observations and concerns related to safety, hazards, escalation, de-escalation of care, and errors in care or the practice environment
- Demonstrates respect for others' perspectives

STANDARD 11 COLLABORATION

The nurse collaborates with the patient, family, and interprofessional team.

COMPETENCIES

- Engages others to promote change, produce optimal outcomes, and enhance patient care
- Adheres to standards that govern behavior among the interprofessional team to create and maintain a healthy work environment
- Partners with the patient, family, and interprofessional team to promote effective and safe transitions across the health care continuum
- Promotes mutual respect, equity, diversity, inclusion, social justice, and engagement among nursing colleagues and the interprofessional team
- Supports other nurses and colleagues through knowledge sharing to provide safe, quality, equitable nursing care

STANDARD 12

LEADERSHIP

The nurse leads in the professional practice setting and the profession.

COMPETENCIES

- Contributes to the creation, application, and maintenance of diverse, equitable, and inclusive healthy work environments
- Supports colleagues through mentoring and other professional development strategies
- Demonstrates the ability to remain patient-centered in a rapidly changing environment
- Directs coordination of care
- Provides oversight of licensed and unlicensed personnel, including delegation of their work
- Contributes expertise to enhance care delivery with involvement on committees, councils, and interprofessional teams
- Advocates for appropriate use of professional association staffing standards
- Advances the profession through participation in professional organizations
- Develops a culture of safety for patients, families, and the interprofessional team
- Promotes communication of information and advancement of the profession through activities such as professional social media participation,[8] writing, publishing, and presentations for professional or lay audiences
- Fosters development and implementation of innovative solutions

STANDARD 13 | EDUCATION

The nurse acquires and maintains evidence-based knowledge and competence to advance their nursing practice.

COMPETENCIES

- Demonstrates accountability for lifelong learning
- Seeks learning opportunities that reflect current and evidence-based nursing competencies in the AACN Synergy Model
- Shares educational findings, experiences, and ideas with peers to elevate progressive care nursing practice
- Engages in formal and informal mentorship
- Fosters a safe and supportive work environment conducive to the professional development of health care professionals
- Considers obtaining professional certification, certificates and credentials, including microcredentials and advanced education
- Maintains professional records or a portfolio that provides evidence of competencies and lifelong learning

STANDARD

14 SCHOLARLY INQUIRY[1]

The nurse integrates scholarly inquiry into practice.

COMPETENCIES

- Inquires about current clinical practices compared with updated evidence for the purpose of providing safe, quality, evidence-based care
- Uses ethical principles to identify clinical problems and formulates clinical questions using evidence generated in a clinical setting, such as patient assessment information and data, outcomes management, and quality-improvement data
- Evaluates evidence to determine applicability to progressive care practice
- Participates in scholarly inquiry through quality improvement, process improvement, and research activities, taking into consideration patient and family beliefs, values, and preferences
- Integrates evidence into policies, procedures, and guidelines
- Implements practice changes based on evidence, clinical expertise, individual patient preferences, and social determinants of health
- Evaluates outcomes of evidence-based decisions and practice changes for individuals, groups, and populations
- Disseminates information regarding best practices supported by evidence
- Participates in activities and strategies to sustain an evidence-based-practice culture
- Demonstrates the value of nursing care in meeting quality, safety, equitable, and cost-effective outcomes

STANDARD 15

QUALITY OF PRACTICE

The nurse contributes to the quality and effectiveness of nursing practice.

COMPETENCIES

- Collaborates with colleagues, subject matter experts, and identified interested parties to promote safe, effective, efficient, equitable, timely, and person-centered evidence-based changes in nursing practice[1]
- Evaluates practice of progressive care nursing in an ongoing manner
- Addresses barriers to quality care and equitable patient outcomes
- Collaborates in the development, implementation, evaluation, and revision of organizational policies, procedures, and/or guidelines
- Uses creativity and innovation to enhance quality nursing care
- Demonstrates quality by documenting application of the nursing process in a responsible, accountable, and ethical manner, and in a clear and retrievable format

STANDARD 16 PROFESSIONAL PRACTICE EVALUATION

The nurse evaluates their own and others' nursing practice.

COMPETENCIES

- Engages in ongoing self-evaluation and reflective practice
- Identifies areas of strength and areas that optimize professional growth
- Identifies gaps in knowledge, competency, and application of nursing practice
- Obtains feedback regarding nursing practice
- Provides peers with formal or informal constructive feedback for improvement
- Takes action to achieve goals identified in the evaluation process

STANDARD 17 RESOURCE STEWARDSHIP

The nurse uses appropriate resources to plan, provide, and sustain services that are safe, effective, and ethically and fiscally responsible.

COMPETENCIES

- Assesses individual patient needs and required, cost-effective resources
- Delegates appropriate elements of care to the correct individual based on assessed needs, condition, and safety of the patient
- Assists the patient and family in identifying and securing appropriate services to address health-related needs
- Informs the patient and family of the options, alternatives, potential complications, and benefits of nursing interventions
- Advocates for additional resources that enhance and support nursing practice, patient safety, and quality of care
- Integrates strategies to address health care disparities and the impact on resource allocation

STANDARD

18 ENVIRONMENTAL HEALTH

The nurse maintains a safe and healthy work environment.

COMPETENCIES

- Embraces implementation of *AACN Standards for Establishing and Sustaining Healthy Work Environments*[6] as a personal and professional obligation
- Role models application of the healthy work environment standards
- Generates enthusiasm among colleagues for the creation of a healthy work environment
- Identifies potentially harmful behaviors that create an unhealthy work environment
- Holds others accountable for maintaining safe work environments
- Takes necessary actions to prevent, mitigate, and address actual and potential environmental risks that may compromise the safety of patients, families, and the interprofessional team
- Minimizes environmental risk factors that may cause physical, emotional, spiritual, and psychological harm or injury to self or others
- Implements strategies to reduce the impact of environmental factors, such as alarm fatigue and disrupted sleep,[9] that jeopardize nurse and patient safety
- Communicates environmental health risks and exposure-reduction strategies to patients, families, and colleagues
- Uses products or treatments consistent with evidence-based practice to reduce environmental threats
- Provides education to patients and families to support population health (eg, immunizations, infection prevention)

STANDARD 18 ENVIRONMENTAL HEALTH (CONT'D)

The nurse maintains a safe and healthy work environment.

- Participates in strategies and activities to promote healthy communities
- Acknowledges their role in disaster preparedness, response, and recovery (natural and manmade)
- Engages in disaster preparation, response, and recovery planning efforts to ensure readiness

REFERENCES

1. American Nurses Association. *Nursing: Scope and Standards of Practice.* 4th ed. American Nurses Association; 2021.

2. American Nurses Association. *Code of Ethics for Nurses with Interpretive Statements.* Nursesbooks.org; 2015.

3. American Association of Critical-Care Nurses. About AACN. Accessed March 11, 2024. https://www.aacn.org/about-aacn

4. National Academies of Sciences, Engineering, and Medicine. *The Future of Nursing 2020-2030: Charting a Path to Achieve Health Equity.* National Academies Press; 2021. https://nap.nationalacademies.org/read/25982/chapter/1#:~:text=Suggested%20Citation%3A%22Front%20Matter.,DC%3A%20The%20National%20Academies%20Press

5. The Joint Commission. R3 Report Issue 30: Workplace violence prevention standards. Accessed August 13, 2024. https://www.jointcommission.org/standards/r3-report/r3-report-issue-30-workplace-violence-prevention-standards/

6. Barden C, ed. *AACN Standards for Establishing and Sustaining Healthy Work Environments: A Journey to Excellence.* 2nd ed. American Association of Critical-Care Nurses; 2016. https://www.aacn.org/nursing-excellence/standards/aacn-standards-for-establishing-and-sustaining-healthy-work-environments

7. The Joint Commission. 8 tips for high-quality handoffs. Accessed June 11, 2024. https://www.jointcommission.org/-/media/tjc/documents/resources/patient-safety-topics/sentinel-event/sea_8_steps_hand_off_infographic_2018pdf.pdf

8. Wells SK. Do's and don'ts of social media use for nursing professionals. Accessed June 11, 2024. https://www.aacn.org/blog/dos-and-donts-of-social-media-use-for-nursing-professionals

9. Bosma S, Christopher R. Implementing a unit-based alarm management bundle for critical care nurses. *Crit Care Nurse.* 2023;43(2):36–45.

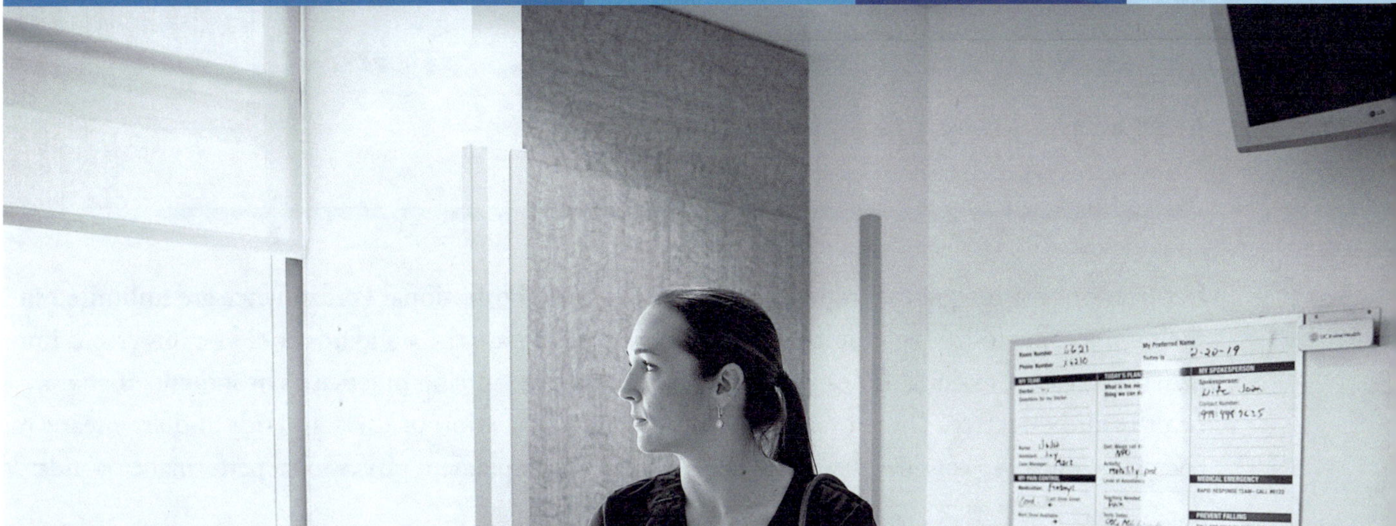
UCI Health

EXAMPLES OF HOW TO INTEGRATE STANDARDS OF PROFESSIONAL PERFORMANCE

Implications for integration and use of the Standards of Professional Performance are unlimited in their scope. The following examples reflect the potential ways the standards could be integrated into activities that are essential for establishing progressive care nursing practice environments that are healthy and effective. These examples demonstrate application of the standards and are meant to encourage nurses to consider these and other strategies to implement professional performance standards.

These vignettes provide examples of how the Standards of Professional Performance competencies are demonstrated in progressive care nursing practice.

STANDARD OF PROFESSIONAL PERFORMANCE 7 – ETHICS COMPETENCIES ARE DEMONSTRATED IN THE FOLLOWING VIGNETTE.

Standard 7: Ethics - The nurse integrates ethics into all aspects of practice.

COMPETENCIES

Ethical accountability to self and patient

To self:

- Demonstrates a commitment to self-care and self-advocacy
- Recognizes moral distress, burnout, and/or compassion fatigue in self and others
- Seeks appropriate support and resources to address moral distress, burnout, and compassion fatigue
- Seeks appropriate resources and support to address personal beliefs and values, biases, and cultural values that may affect ethical obligations to patients

- Promotes the development and sustainment of a healthy work environment
- Shows zero tolerance for workplace violence,[5] including bullying, verbal abuse, discrimination, and incivility[6]

To patient:

- Contributes to resolving ethical issues involving the patient, family, and interprofessional team
- Questions health care practice when necessary for safety and quality improvement
- Maintains respect for patient autonomy, dignity, values, beliefs, and rights at all times

ETHICS VIGNETTE #1

A progressive care nurse admitted an older adult patient who is detoxing from alcohol and who had severe withdrawal symptoms, including tremors, hallucinations, and an extreme headache clouding judgment. The patient became more irritable as the night continued with the progressive care nurse doing frequent rounding for their safety and to appropriately score them on the Clinical Institute Withdrawal Assessment (CIWA) scale. The patient became increasingly agitated, escalating from brief verbal comments to physical violence. The patient was placed in 4-point restraints. The progressive care nurse had emotional and physical injuries related to the actions and was unsure what the next steps should be. It was not clear if the nurse could do anything due to the patient not being aware of their actions, as confusion and withdrawal clouded their judgment. The nurse came forward to the unit manager about these concerns regarding reporting patients under the influence. By using the organizational zero-tolerance policy, the physical and verbal incident with the patient was reported for the safety of this progressive care nurse and future nurses. The unit manager offered more resources to support the progressive care nurse's mental health and created a new hospital strategy for increased security rounding on withdrawal patients to mitigate and prevent the risk of verbal, emotional, and physical attacks against staff. The hospital also created ongoing education and training to create a safe culture and inform staff to always report workplace violence incidents to help with future cases.

STANDARD OF PROFESSIONAL PERFORMANCE 7 – ETHICS COMPETENCIES ARE DEMONSTRATED IN THE FOLLOWING VIGNETTE. (CONT'D)

Standard 7: Ethics - The nurse integrates ethics into all aspects of practice.

COMPETENCIES

Ethical accountability to patient

- Practices as guided by ANA's *Code of Ethics for Nurses with Interpretive Statements*[2] and AACN's core values[3]
- Promotes ethical accountability and integrity in relationships, patient confidentiality and privacy, organizational decisions, and stewardship of resources in consideration of the dynamic nature of care transitions and patient acuity
- Advocates for the concerns of the patient, family, and community
- Supports the patient and family in self-determination and informed decision making
- Maintains respect for patient autonomy, dignity, values, beliefs, and rights at all times
- Delivers care in an inclusive, equitable, culturally, and psychologically safe manner that meets the diverse needs of the patient, family, and community
- Uses available resources in making ethical decisions

ETHICS VIGNETTE #2

A progressive care nurse was taking care of an older patient who was fighting complicated pneumonia and pancreatic cancer. The patient was given an unknown amount of time to live. The patient's family was determined for the patient to return home with their significant other, independent with no limitations. The patient's condition was declining as the hospital stay continued, with increased work of breathing and increased oxygen needs. The patient voiced to the nurse how wonderful a life they had lived with a wonderful family and significant other, but the patient was getting very tired of all the tests and medications.

The nurse could see how tired the patient was getting and wanted the patient to be comfortable with as little pain as possible. The progressive care nurse was struggling with how to support the family's decision when they knew that the outlook for the patient was not promising. The nurse reached out to the primary care physician, asking if there could be a care conference with all the physicians overseeing the patient's care and the family to help find potential solutions to the patient's complex circumstances.

The family appreciated the nurse advocating for the patient, who was unaware of how complex their health expectations looked. Because the patient was still decisional, they came together as a family and treatment team to work out what was best for the patient, and the patient and family were able to make an informed decision about care.

ETHICS VIGNETTE #3

Two progressive care nurses were working the night shift together and had wanted to attempt a new video trend on social media that other nurses had been trying out. They were not aware of the hospital's social media policies or considering their work surroundings. They created a video with their badges on, and in the background, there was a patient's last name and side profile in view. The charge nurse for the shift saw them in action and reminded them that it is not professionally appropriate to make videos at work. This video was a patient privacy breach and could flag the hospital for a privacy violation. The charge nurse reminded them that nurses have a responsibility to protect patient confidentiality and respect boundaries. The 2 nurses indicated an understanding of the situation and removed the post as it was unprofessional and against hospital policy. They took it as a good learning lesson for new nurses and created an educational poster for the hospital about being aware of their surroundings, the use of social media, and how it could negatively impact patients and families if used in an unprofessional manner.

REFERENCES

American Association of Critical-Care Nurses. AACN core values. Accessed August 1, 2024. https://www.aacn.org/about-aacn

American Nurses Association. *Nursing: Scope and Standards of Practice.* 4th ed. Nursingworld.org; 2021.

American Nurses Association. *Code of Ethics for Nurses with Interpretive Statements.* Nursesbooks.org; 2015.

STANDARD OF PROFESSIONAL PERFORMANCE 8 – ADVOCACY COMPETENCIES ARE DEMONSTRATED IN THE FOLLOWING VIGNETTE.

Standard 8: Advocacy - The nurse demonstrates advocacy in all roles and settings.

COMPETENCIES

- Promotes patient preferences while preserving patients' dignity and rights while involving them in the shared decision-making process
- Advocates for equitable and appropriate resources that enhance and support nursing practice, patient safety, and quality of care
- Champions the allocation of resources specific to the patient's needs to support outcomes beyond hospitalization
- Serves as a voice for vulnerable populations, advocating for policies and interventions that promote health equity
- Advocates for escalation of care based on the needs of the patient

ADVOCACY VIGNETTE

An older adult patient was experiencing abdominal pain and hematuria that had been increasing over the last several weeks. The patient went to the local community hospital where imaging revealed a large mass, while lab work revealed a hemoglobin of 6.3 g/dL and a creatinine of 8.1 mg/dL. The patient was admitted to the oncology PCU for further workup and treatment planning. The hospitalist consulted a gynecologic oncologist, as the patient was diagnosed with stage IV cervical cancer with a large mass compressing the right kidney.

On day 2 of the patient's hospital stay, the oncologist rounded with the progressive care nurse, the patient, and the family. After reviewing the imaging and lab work, the oncologist felt that little could be done and told the patient that they likely had less than 3 months to live. The patient remained very quiet throughout the visit after the physician left. Later, the nurse sat with the patient to offer support and see what questions the patient might have now that they had some time to digest the news. The patient stated they were scared and did not want to accept the prognosis. The patient asked the nurse what else they could do.

The nurse called the physician to advocate for the patient and arranged a family meeting. The patient advocate assisted the nurse in setting a time that the patient, family, oncologist, and nephrologist could meet to review the case. To prepare for this meeting, the nurse advised the patient to consider their questions and write them down to serve as a guide for the discussion. It allowed the patient time to process the diagnosis and ask questions so the entire care team could be on the same page.

During the meeting, the patient voiced their questions and concerns to the oncologist and stated that they had heard of new treatment options that might be available at the academic medical center downtown. The oncologist was able to discuss the case with the surgical oncology team there, and it was deemed the patient was a candidate for continued treatment. To prepare for the transfer, the team discussed with the patient the plan to place a nephrostomy tube to relieve the compressed kidney, in addition to the hemodialysis that was started on admission. The patient agreed with this plan and once the nephrostomy tube was placed, the patient was able to transfer to the academic medical center. At the center, treatment including chemotherapy, and radiation was started to shrink the tumor with the eventual plan to remove the mass. The nurse who advocated for a meeting where the patient was able to ask questions and be a part of their health care discussion helped the patient feel empowered.

EXAMPLES

STANDARD OF PROFESSIONAL PERFORMANCE 9 – RESPECTFUL AND EQUITABLE PRACTICE COMPETENCIES ARE DEMONSTRATED IN THE FOLLOWING VIGNETTE.

Standard 9: Respectful and Equitable Practice - The nurse practices with cultural humility and inclusiveness.

COMPETENCIES

- Identifies opportunities for lifelong learning to understand values, beliefs, heritage, cultural preferences, worldviews, choices, unconscious biases, and decision-making processes of self, peers, and population served
- Identifies skills and tools needed for the specific culture, literacy, and language of the progressive care population served

A nurse working in a PCU that cares for patients with substance use disorder wants to learn how to advocate and better care for them. What was the plan?

RESPECTFUL AND EQUITABLE PRACTICE VIGNETTE

A nurse is working in a progressive care unit (PCU) that cares for people with substance use disorder (SUD). The nurse notices how these patients are often treated differently and stigmatized by other staff members and knows this doesn't align with the nursing ethics that were taught in school. The nurse also personally knows individuals who have struggled with addiction and the ability to receive equitable care, and the nurse feels uncomfortable with what they're observing.

Wanting to learn how to better care for this patient population and advocate for them, the nurse approaches the unit's nursing leadership to ask if there is anything that can be done. The unit educator connects the nurse to a 4-hour anti-stigma course that the intensive care unit (ICU) incorporated into their nurse residency program. The course consisted of presentations from experts and people with lived experiences, as well as role play, demonstration, and electronic resources throughout the program. The course had an overall positive effect on attendees' therapeutic attitudes and perceived stigma toward people with SUD. The course also helped the learners recognize their own biases and what strategies can help reduce the impact those biases may have on the care they give.

The nurse returns to their unit and shares the experience with nursing leadership, who invite the nurse to share more in a staff meeting. The nurse presents a 5-minute summary of the workshop to colleagues, and many express interest in also attending the course. The ICU and PCU educators collaborated to develop shared education between the 2 departments, which led to more nurse champions for people with SUD in both units. The success of this strategy to promote health equity reached the chief nursing officer, who decided to roll out this course hospital-wide. Over the next year, therapeutic attitudes and perceived stigma were evaluated and showed improvement.

In the PCU, the nurse noticed a culture shift toward more compassionate care for those with SUD, and nurses in the unit felt more empowered to speak up when they noticed behavior or overheard conversations that didn't align with ethical values and equitable care for all patients.

REFERENCE

Dion K, Griggs S. Teaching those who care how to care for a person with substance use disorder. *Nurse Educ.* 2020;45(6):321–325. https://doi.org/10.1097/NNE.0000000000000808

STANDARD OF PROFESSIONAL PERFORMANCE 10 – COMMUNICATION COMPETENCIES ARE DEMONSTRATED IN THE FOLLOWING VIGNETTE.

Standard 10: Communication - The nurse communicates effectively in all areas of practice.

COMPETENCIES

- Minimizes risks associated with patient handoffs, transfers, and transitions of care
- Conveys accurate information to patients, families, and the interprofessional team in a way they can understand
- Confirms communication is heard and the message is understood
- Validates own understanding of the rationale for care processes and decisions
- Clarifies the rationale for care processes and decisions with others, as appropriate
- Contributes professional nursing perspective in discussions with the interprofessional team
- Follows the chain of command to report observations and concerns related to safety, hazards, escalation, de-escalation of care, and errors in care or the practice environment
- Demonstrates respect for others' perspectives

Skilled communication is an essential element in promoting respectful peer collaboration and a culture of safety and equity. Following is an example that reflects integration of this standard:

COMMUNICATION VIGNETTE

Rey is currently working in a 16-bed PCU. He is very hardworking and recognized by his peers as compassionate. Two patients that Rey is treating are transferring to medical-surgical. In preparation, Rey knows he needs to make sure Mr Smith's and Ms Gonzalez's conditions and future needs are clearly reported to the accepting nurse and all handoffs are complete for their care, medical reviews, and belongings. As Rey was planning the transfer of Mr Smith, Rey assessed that the patient would probably need a heparin drip prior to transfer. Rey requested the heparin drip from the pharmacy. As Rey was busy transferring Ms Gonzalez, he noticed that the heparin drip for Mr Smith was nearly empty. Rey called the pharmacy to ensure the heparin was prepared so that it would be ready and available before transferring Mr Smith.

The heparin drip was delivered on time, because Rey communicated early and anticipated the time medication should be given. After Rey connected the heparin to the patient, he prepared an SBAR (Situation, Background, Assessment, and Recommendation) sheet. Rey then called the accepting nurse to give report. As the final step of the verbal report, Rey asked the nurse, "What questions do you have?"

Rey asked the receiving nurse to make sure the room was ready prior to transfer. After Rey transferred Mr Smith to medical-surgical and returned to the PCU, Rey noticed that the hospitalist resident had entered an order to stop the heparin drip on the just-transferred patient. Rey messaged the hospitalist resident. Upon confirmation of the order, Rey questioned the resident about the order for discontinuation, citing the patient's past history of renal stenosis and occlusion. The resident confirmed the discontinuation order. Rey called the medical-surgical nurse who received Mr Smith to ensure that they were aware of the resident's verbal order to stop heparin.

The medical-surgical nurse and Rey were both concerned about discontinuation of the heparin, because they were aware of the patient's history and the procedures for bilateral renal stenosis and occlusion. At this point, the medical-surgical nurse called the attending cardiologist supervising the resident and, using the CUS (concerned, uncomfortable, safety) mnemonic, asked for order clarification:

- "I am **c**oncerned that the patient, Mr Smith, has a history of renal stenosis and occlusion.
- I am **u**ncomfortable that the hospitalist resident discontinued the heparin drip.
- I think this is a **s**afety issue for the patient due to his history of occlusion."

The cardiologist agreed with the nurse's assessment and gave the order to continue the heparin drip. The cardiologist also assured the nurse that they would follow up with the hospitalist resident to ensure the resident is aware of the order change and provide explanation for the reason to maintain the heparin infusion.

Since Rey gave a complete SBAR report to the receiving medical-surgical nurse, the receiving nurse was aware of the patient's situation, and they prevented the patient from a potentially dangerous complication.

EXAMPLES

STANDARD OF PROFESSIONAL PERFORMANCE 11 – COLLABORATION COMPETENCIES DEMONSTRATED IN THE FOLLOWING VIGNETTE.

Standard 11: Collaboration - The nurse collaborates with the patient, family, and interprofessional team.

COMPETENCIES

- Engages others to promote change, produce optimal outcomes, and enhance patient care
- Adheres to standards that govern behavior among the interprofessional team to create and maintain a healthy work environment
- Partners with the patient, family, and interprofessional team to promote effective and safe transitions across the health care continuum
- Promotes mutual respect, equity, diversity, inclusion, social justice, and engagement among nursing colleagues and the interprofessional team
- Supports other nurses and colleagues through knowledge sharing to provide safe, quality, equitable nursing care

COLLABORATION VIGNETTE

A progressive care nurse working in a 500-bed academic teaching hospital noticed that continuous positive airway pressure (CPAP) treatment had not been ordered for a patient who was admitted to the hospital due to a hypertensive crisis. This patient had an existing diagnosis of obstructive sleep apnea (OSA). For over 2 weeks of hospitalization, this patient continued to have labile blood pressure.

The nurse remembered coming across literature discussing OSA as a cause of secondary hypertension. The nurse also discovered that the patient was prescribed CPAP for home management of OSA but stated "my CPAP lives in my closet collecting dust." The nurse reviewed the literature and consulted with primary medical team colleagues, determining that managing OSA might be beneficial in the setting of acute hypertension. The nurse and the primary medical team then discussed the benefits of using CPAP with the patient, consulted with the respiratory team, and initiated CPAP treatment for the patient.

The nurse consulted with the patient proactively to identify barriers to using CPAP at home. The patient indicated that discomfort with the CPAP mask was a major issue. The nurse then ensured this crucial information was given to a sleep specialist when a referral was made by the primary medical team. Upon hospital discharge, the nurse included educational materials on OSA and outpatient sleep referral information in the discharge package.

STANDARD OF PROFESSIONAL PERFORMANCE 12 – LEADERSHIP COMPETENCIES DEMONSTRATED IN THE FOLLOWING VIGNETTE.

Standard 12: Leadership - The nurse leads in the professional practice setting and the profession.

COMPETENCIES

- Contributes expertise to enhance care delivery with involvement on committees, councils, and interprofessional teams
- Advocates for appropriate use of professional association staffing standards
- Advances the profession through participation in professional organizations
- Develops a culture of safety for patients, families, and the interprofessional team
- Fosters development and implementation of innovative solutions

LEADERSHIP VIGNETTE

After 2 years in a progressive care unit (PCU), a nurse is asked by their nurse manager to represent the unit by participating in the hospital's Nursing Practice Council (NPC). The hospital understands the importance of Healthy Work Environment (HWE) Standards and uses this council to enhance true collaboration across the clinical areas. They know that an HWE leads to improved patient safety and nurse retention.

At one of the first meetings, the PCU nurse listens to an intensive care unit (ICU) nurse on the council share that they recently attended the National Teaching Institute & Critical Care Exposition (NTI), where they heard about the American Association of Critical-Care Nurses' *AACN Standards for Appropriate Staffing in Adult Critical Care.* The ICU nurse explains that, while it's specific to adult critical care, this document could be a good place to start to develop their own organizational and unit-specific staffing guidelines, because many of the standards apply to most clinical environments. The group creates a subcommittee of critical care and progressive care nurses who are tasked to familiarize themselves with the document, look for areas where they may already be aligned and areas of opportunity, and report back to the group.

Over the next month, the PCU nurse spends time thoroughly reviewing AACN's appropriate staffing guidelines and recommendations, while taking time to understand the rationale behind them. They educate themselves on the potential consequences of inadequate staffing, such as increased patient mortality rates, higher rates of nurse burnout, and compromised quality of care.

Over the next several months, the NPC continues to devote time and attention to this topic and begins collaborating with nursing leadership. The PCU nurse is one of the individuals who is able to present the findings to the Nursing Management Council for their input and guidance. The leadership group listens and shows understanding about how important appropriate staffing is to the patients and to the nurses who work in the units and how it can lead to higher job satisfaction, lower staff turnover, higher patient and family satisfaction, and better patient outcomes. Working closely with facility partners (direct care nurses, ancillary staff, providers, budget and legal advisors, senior leadership, etc), they use these guidelines to develop a pilot for an enhanced staffing approach in the ICU. They intend to implement the guidelines, track data, and evaluate the outcomes of the intervention. The next steps include continuing this work and developing similar guidelines for the PCU and other units.

The PCU nurse's individual contributions were vital, because they could represent their unit and share the unique struggles and staffing concerns that they've witnessed over the last 2 years. The NPC's work was an essential step toward beginning to meet the first standard of appropriate staffing by having direct care nurses participate in all aspects of staffing: planning, implementation, and evaluation.

REFERENCE

American Association of Critical-Care Nurses. *AACN Standards for Appropriate Staffing in Adult Critical Care.* https://www.aacn.org/nursing-excellence/standards/aacn-standards-for-appropriate-staffing-in-adult-critical-care

EXAMPLES

STANDARD OF PROFESSIONAL PERFORMANCE 13 – EDUCATION COMPETENCIES DEMONSTRATED IN THE FOLLOWING VIGNETTE.

Standard 13: Education - The nurse acquires and maintains evidence-based knowledge and competence to advance their nursing practice.

COMPETENCIES

- Shares educational findings, experiences, and ideas with peers to elevate progressive care nursing practice
- Engages in formal and informal mentorship
- Fosters a safe and supportive work environment conducive to the professional development of health care professionals

EDUCATION VIGNETTE

A progressive care registered nurse (RN), Zoe, with 8 years of nursing experience, was working on a high-acuity 28-bed cardiac surgical stepdown unit beside a newer RN, Jeff, with 3 years of medical-surgical nursing experience, who had just transferred to the cardiac surgical stepdown unit a few months ago. Jeff was 3 weeks off orientation but was visibly overwhelmed with the acuity of the patients in cardiac surgical stepdown. Zoe noticed Jeff running between rooms and struggling with finding appropriate supplies quickly, leading him to go in and out of rooms multiple times, which seemed to contribute to his feeling of being behind.

When Jeff was finished administering morning medications to his 4 patients, Zoe asked Jeff if he was available for a quick chat. Zoe and Jeff went into the team conference room, and Zoe asked Jeff how his shift was going. Jeff admitted he was extremely overwhelmed with the patients' acuity, and he was still adjusting to the increased potential for decompensation of the unit's patient population. Jeff expressed feeling supported by the charge nurse but admitted that he felt like he was constantly bothering them with questions. Zoe acknowledged and validated Jeff's feelings of being overwhelmed and assured Jeff that he was not a bother to the charge nurse. Zoe told him that he could also use her as a resource for any questions. Zoe also offered to share strategies that she tries to use during her shift with clustering care, prioritizing the tasks she must complete early in the shift such as full assessments, medication administrations, and dressing changes, and identifying the tasks she must complete by the end of her shift but aren't as high priority. Zoe offered to walk Jeff through the unit again, acknowledging the significant amount of information a nurse receives during orientation and verbalizing that this new walk-through could be with fresh eyes.

Jeff was eager to hear Zoe's work strategies and grateful to be reoriented to the unit's space and supplies with new knowledge and perspective. Zoe walked Jeff through the unit, showing him where to find the most commonly used wound care and dressing supplies, where the chest tube supplies and thoracic cart for new chest tube insertions were stored, the location of replacement wires for the bedside physiologic monitors, and where to look for the walkers for ambulating patients. Zoe shared how she organizes the information she receives from report to set up her shift for success. At the conclusion of their interaction, Jeff and Zoe went back to their individual patient assignments, but Zoe witnessed Jeff seeming less flustered, accomplishing his tasks and providing care in a more efficient fashion.

While Zoe is a preceptor on the unit, she was not assigned as Jeff's preceptor during his orientation. She recognized that Jeff needed additional support after orientation. Zoe leveraged her many years of cardiac surgical stepdown nursing experience, as well as her mentorship experience as a preceptor to new graduate and experienced nurses, and went out of her way to offer support to a colleague while on shift. Zoe taught Jeff essential skills of clustering tasks for efficient care delivery, advised Jeff on the most common equipment necessary for success, and offered tips on organizing information after report to create a successful shift. Most of all, Zoe offered Jeff validation of his feelings and supported him as a nurse in a new environment.

STANDARD OF PROFESSIONAL PERFORMANCE 14 – SCHOLARLY INQUIRY COMPETENCIES ARE DEMONSTRATED IN THE FOLLOWING VIGNETTE.

Standard 14: Scholarly Inquiry - The nurse integrates scholarly inquiry into practice.

COMPETENCIES

- Inquires about current clinical practices compared with updated evidence for the purpose of providing safe, quality, evidence-based care
- Uses ethical principles to identify clinical problems and formulates clinical questions using evidence generated in a clinical setting, such as patient assessment information and data, outcomes management, and quality-improvement data
- Evaluates evidence to determine applicability to progressive care nursing practice
- Participates in scholarly inquiry through quality improvement, process improvement, and research activities, taking into consideration patient and family beliefs, values, and preferences
- Integrates evidence into policies, procedures, and guidelines
- Implements practice changes based on evidence, clinical expertise, individual patient preferences, and social determinants of health
- Evaluates outcomes of evidence-based decisions and practice changes for individuals, groups, and populations
- Disseminates information regarding best practices supported by evidence
- Participates in activities and strategies to sustain an evidence-based-practice culture
- Demonstrates the value of nursing care in meeting quality, safety, equitable, and cost-effective outcomes

SCHOLARLY INQUIRY VIGNETTE

A progressive care nurse noticed that hospital-wide policies were often outdated and not updated in a timely manner, because clinical nurse specialists are often stretched thin. The nurse was concerned that policies with outdated evidence may not provide bedside nurses with evidence-based guidance in nursing practice. Therefore, the nurse brought their observations to the Unit Based Council (UPC). The UPC then asked the nurse to bring their assessment to the Local Practice Council (LPC). The nurse spoke with the LPC, took the lead, and formed a policy and procedure work group with several other nurses. The policy and procedure work group was granted project time to work on reviewing literature and make recommendations on revisions to nursing policies. The nurse-led policy and procedure work group not only encourages shared governance initiatives but also supports evidence-based changes.

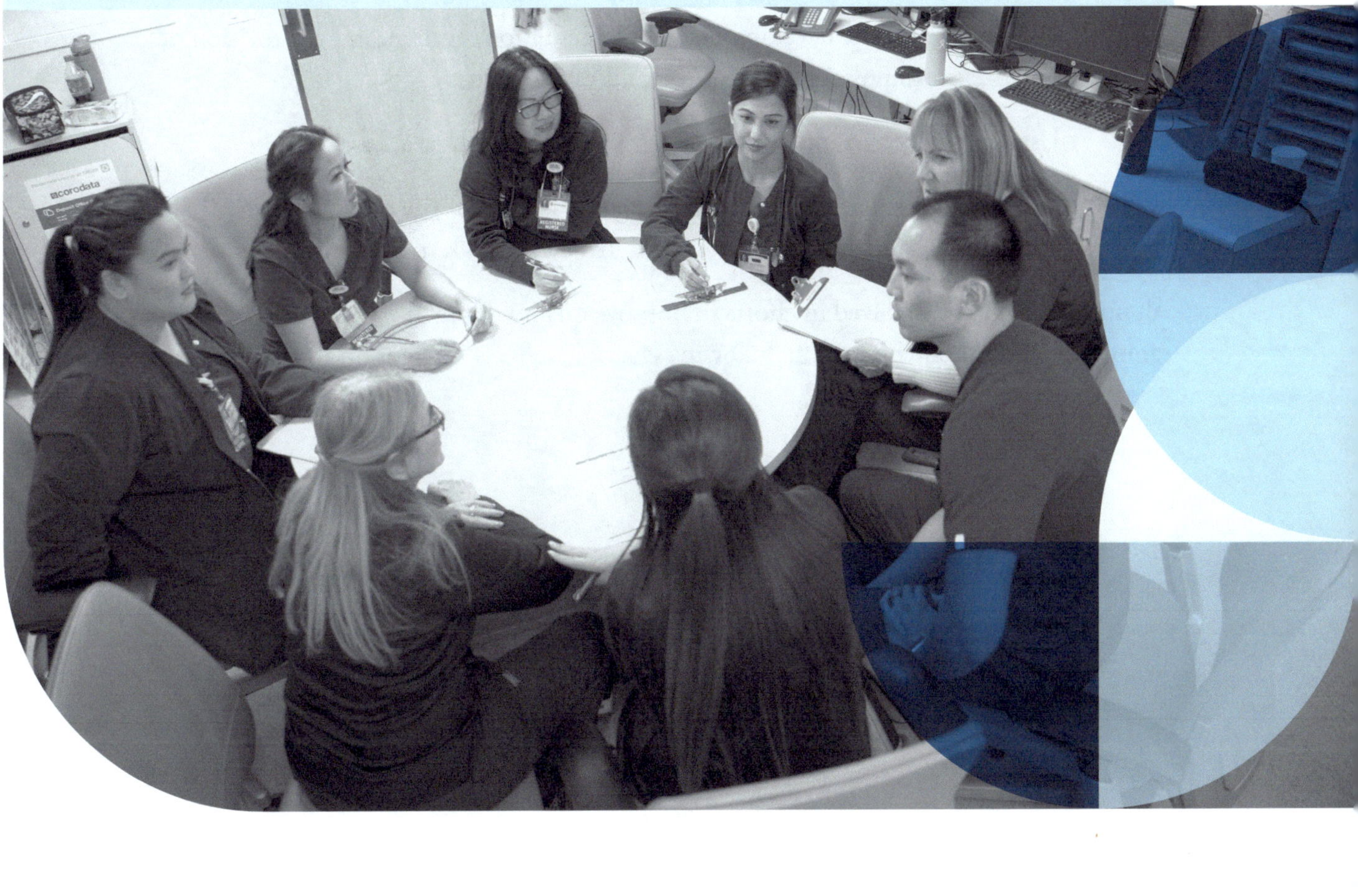

STANDARD OF PROFESSIONAL PERFORMANCE 15 – QUALITY OF PRACTICE COMPETENCIES ARE DEMONSTRATED IN THE FOLLOWING VIGNETTE.

Standard 15: Quality of Practice - The nurse contributes to the quality and effectiveness of nursing practice.

COMPETENCIES

- Collaborates with colleagues, subject matter experts, and identified interested parties to promote safe, effective, efficient, equitable, timely, and person-centered evidence-based changes in nursing practice[1]
- Evaluates practice of progressive care nursing in an ongoing manner
- Addresses barriers to quality care and equitable patient outcomes
- Collaborates in the development, implementation, evaluation, and revision of organizational policies, procedures, and/or guidelines
- Uses creativity and innovation to enhance quality nursing care
- Demonstrates quality by documenting application of the nursing process in a responsible, accountable, and ethical manner, and in a clear and retrievable format

All nurses need to be involved in efforts to improve quality of practice, patient, clinician and workplace safety, and clinical outcomes. The following example reflects integration of this standard:

QUALITY OF PRACTICE VIGNETTE

A progressive care unit (PCU) nurse working in a 200-bed community hospital noticed that the facility's established sepsis protocol was not routinely ordered when patients were admitted into the PCU with a diagnosis of sepsis. As a result, the care provided for these patients varied widely with equally variable outcomes.

The nurse reviewed current literature and available screening technology and consulted with several physician colleagues, determining the protocol was outdated and too rigid to provide equitable, patient-centered care. The nurse initiated a medical-record review of patients with sepsis in order to identify similar patient characteristics and any deficiencies or inconsistencies in care delivery. The review revealed consistent care for patients triaged through the emergency department but very little active screening of patients already admitted to inpatient units.

The nurse consulted with staff to identify barriers to routine screening and early identification of these patients. Working closely with the progressive care team, medical provider staff, antibiotic stewardship committee, nursing informatics, nursing leadership, pharmacy, and diversity, equity, and inclusion (DEI) committee, information technology (IT), and a small team of champions from each inpatient unit, the nurse developed an updated sepsis screening and treatment protocol that included automatic triggers and electronic notification of staff when screening criteria was met; it reflected the current best evidence for equitable clinical management of each patient. The nurse also developed a visual screening tool and extended education beyond the inpatient units to include all outpatient services on campus that are served by the facility's rapid response team. The nurse continues to monitor the program through equity, quality, and mortality data on a quarterly basis.

STANDARD OF PROFESSIONAL PERFORMANCE 16 – PROFESSIONAL PRACTICE EVALUATION COMPETENCIES ARE DEMONSTRATED IN THE FOLLOWING VIGNETTE.

Standard 16: Professional Practice Evaluation - The nurse evaluates their own and others' nursing practice.

COMPETENCIES

- Engages in ongoing self-evaluation and reflective practice
- Identifies areas of strength and areas that optimize professional growth
- Identifies gaps in knowledge, competency, and application of nursing practice
- Obtains feedback regarding nursing practice
- Provides peers with formal or informal constructive feedback for improvement
- Takes action to achieve goals identified in the evaluation process

PROFESSIONAL PRACTICE EVALUATION VIGNETTE

Individual performance measurement and improvement are as important as unit- or hospital-based process improvement. Strategies that reflect integration of this standard include the following example:

Asher is a new nurse starting on a stepdown unit at a small community hospital. Since they are a novice, they are asked to conduct a self-evaluation of their performance after 6 months.

Their mentor recommended *AACN Scope and Standards of Professional Practice and Performance* and *AACN Competence Framework for Progressive and Critical Care: Initial Competency 2022* as the frameworks for self-evaluation. Professional Performance Standard 14, Scholarly Inquiry, matches well with the synergy competency of clinical judgment. Asher identifies key elements required to provide care and consistently follows evidence-based-practice protocols. Their decision making includes recognizing scope of practice, and they know how to mobilize resources in an emergency. As a new nurse, they were able to document the assessment, plan, interventions, and patient's response.

In self-reflection on the *caring practices* competency, they recognize their strength to create a compassionate and supportive environment. They display the *advocacy* competency and standard of performance of *ethics* with their ability to represent the concerns of the family and the rights of the patient. The *synergy* competency and standard of performance of *collaboration* can be assessed with the *communication* standard of performance. *Collaboration* and *communication* were demonstrated when they participated in team meetings and communicated patient data with other disciplines pertinent to quality-improvement projects being discussed. The *synergy* competency of *systems thinking* and the performance standard of *resource utilization* were consistently seen through their awareness of the availability and management of supplies, equipment, and personnel on the unit.

Asher recognizes and adapts their style of education to include the learning needs of the patient and family, exhibiting the *facilitation of learning* competency. Asher is interested in learning and frequently seeks evidence-based resources to answer questions on the best approach to care for critically ill patients, exhibiting the synergy competency of *clinical inquiry* and the standards of performance of *education* and *quality of practice*.

A major strength is their demonstration of sensitivity to diverse cultures, which displays the *response to diversity* competency. An example occurred when a Hmong patient wanted to have a local shaman at the bedside during a procedure. Asher was instrumental in ensuring that this request could be carried out. When evaluating performance using the scope and standards and the AACN Synergy Model, a consistent approach to nursing professionalism is demonstrated, ensuring optimal and equitable patient outcomes.

STANDARD OF PROFESSIONAL PERFORMANCE 17 – RESOURCE STEWARDSHIP COMPETENCIES ARE DEMONSTRATED IN THE FOLLOWING VIGNETTE.

Standard 17: Resource Stewardship - The nurse uses appropriate resources to plan, provide, and sustain services that are safe, effective, and ethically and fiscally responsible.

COMPETENCIES

- Assesses individual patient needs and required, cost-effective resources
- Informs the patient and family of the options, alternatives, risks, potential complications, and benefits of nursing interventions
- Advocates for additional resources that enhance and support nursing practice, patient safety, and quality of care
- Integrates strategies to address health care disparities and the impact on resource allocation

The nurse uses appropriate resources to plan, provide, and sustain services that are safe, effective, and ethically and fiscally responsible.

RESOURCE STEWARDSHIP VIGNETTE

A progressive care nurse is caring for an older adult patient who transferred from the trauma ICU. The patient's history includes being admitted from a skilled nursing facility, status post ground-level fall while ambulating to the bathroom and sustaining an epidural hematoma. While admitting the patient to the progressive care unit, the nurse completes a 2-nurse skin assessment, also known as a 4 eyes skin assessment, to assess for skin breakdown and pressure injuries. The primary nurse educates the patient and family about this nurse-driven intervention to assess for current skin breakdown and pressure injuries and to prevent them from worsening. They inform the patient and family that worsening pressure injuries and skin breakdown can lead to complications, such as longer hospital stays and risk for infection. During the skin assessment, both nurses noticed a stage I pressure injury to the patient's sacrum, so they placed a wound care nurse consult, and the primary nurse placed a protective barrier dressing on the patient's sacrum. Turns were completed every 2 hours, and the bedside nurses collaborated with the wound care nurses to prevent the pressure injury from worsening. Patient and family education was continued as wound care recommendations were provided.

REFERENCE

Singleton E, Jenkins L, Phearman L, Stewart S. Implementation of 4 eyes skin assessment in the pediatric PACU. *J PeriAnesth Nurs*. 2023;38(4):e29. Accessed August 6, 2024. https://doi.org/10.1016/j.jopan.2023.06.030

STANDARD OF PROFESSIONAL PERFORMANCE 18 – ENVIRONMENTAL HEALTH COMPETENCIES ARE DEMONSTRATED IN THE FOLLOWING VIGNETTE.

Standard 18: Environmental Health - The nurse maintains a safe and healthy work environment.

COMPETENCIES

- Takes necessary actions to prevent, mitigate, and address actual and potential environmental risks that may compromise the safety of patients, families, and the interprofessional team
- Minimizes environmental risk factors that may cause physical, emotional, spiritual, and psychological harm or injury to self or others
- Communicates environmental health risks and exposure-reduction strategies to patients, families, and colleagues
- Uses products or treatments consistent with evidence-based practice to reduce environmental threats
- Provides education to patients and families to support population health (eg, immunizations, infection prevention)

Nurses have a responsibility to ensure that care is delivered in a work environment that does not harm the patient and family. In addition, nurses have the right to provide care in a safe, healthy work environment. Environments that consider the well-being of the patient, family, and nurse are established and maintained through interprofessional collaboration. Strategies that reflect integration of this standard include the following example:

ENVIRONMENTAL HEALTH VIGNETTE

A migrant farm worker comes to the emergency department with his family. His family states that he started wheezing after working in the field. His history includes asthma. Symptoms of respiratory distress and bradycardia are noted, noninvasive ventilation is applied, and he is admitted to the progressive care unit (PCU).

The PCU nurse investigates by asking questions about the type of pesticide used in the field and whether there was spraying while he was there. Specific questions include whether the field was wet when they were picking the crop, if he had lunch in the field, and if his job duties include mixing and applying chemicals. His acetylcholinesterase was depressed by 50% of normal, so it was likely he had been exposed to organophosphates.

The nurse was aware of the antidote, atropine, for organophosphate exposure and that dosing could include up to 300 mg/day or a continuous infusion. The nurse was also aware of the adverse effects of atropine toxicity, such as fever, muscle fasciculation, and delirium. The nurse educated her colleagues that the alkyl phosphates and phenols to which organophosphates are hydrolyzed may be detected in urine up to 48 hours after exposure, and nurses attending to the patient should avoid direct contact with heavily contaminated clothing and vomitus.

The nurse was competent in taking an environmental history, familiar with the pesticides used in the local community, and prepared to educate colleagues and treat patients who have conditions associated with pesticide exposure.

REFERENCE

American Nurses Association. *ANA's Principles of Environmental Health for Nursing Practice with Implementation Strategies*. Accessed August 6, 2024. https://www.nursingworld.org/globalassets/docs/ana/ethics/principles-of-environmental-health-online_final.pdf

GLOSSARY

AACN Core Values

- Integrity — Nurses demonstrate sound judgment, ethical behavior, and accountability in all we do.
- Inclusion — Nurses cultivate an inclusive and equitable culture, where everyone contributes their unique strengths and perspectives.
- Transformation — Nurses drive change and innovation to positively impact the health care system and improve the lives of patients, families, and nurses.
- Leadership — Nurses advocate and influence to achieve and sustain optimal outcomes and healthy work environments.
- Relationships — Nurses collaborate and advance partnerships, honoring each individual to strengthen the collective.[1]

AACN Synergy Model for Patient Care – conceptual model of certified progressive and critical care nursing practice that specifies the needs and/or characteristics of patients and families drive the competencies of the nurse from novice through advanced practice[2]

Acuity – referring to the stability of the patient's condition. As the patient becomes more unstable, acuity is said to increase, and as they become more stable, acuity is said to decrease.[3]

Acutely and critically ill or injured patients – patients who are at high risk for complications, secondary injury, or mortality due to present health problems. The more critically ill or injured the patient, the more likely they are to be highly vulnerable, unstable, and complex.

Assessment – systematic, dynamic process by which the nurse, through interaction with the patient/family, nursing personnel, and interprofessional team, collects and analyzes data. Data may include the following dimensions: physical, psychological, social, environmental, regulatory, external, cultural, cognitive, functional, organizational, developmental, and economic.

Burnout syndrome – signs and symptoms of exhaustion, depersonalization, and reduced personal accomplishment triggered by a discrepancy between the employee's expectations and ideas of the role and the actual demands and expectations of the job[4]

Caregiver (paid/unpaid) – member of a person's social network who assists with the activities of daily living. Caregiving is usually for individuals who are minors or those with a disability, a disease, or a mental disorder.[5]

Compassion fatigue – negative aspect of helping those who experience traumatic stress and suffering that is often linked to burnout; a related concept in which the nurse experiences slowly developing frustration, a loss of control, and generally low morale[4]

Competence – performs successfully at an expected level. Competent nurses can be influenced by the nature of the situation, which includes consideration of the setting, resources, and person.[6]

Competency – expected level of performance that integrates knowledge, skills and abilities (KSAs), and judgment[6]

Competency-based orientation – learner focused, it is based on the attainment of established competencies. The assessment of the learner determines individual orientation.[7]

Confidentiality – protection of medical and health information to remain private

Continuity of care – interprofessional process that includes patients and families/significant others in the development of a coordinated plan; a process that facilitates the patient's transition between settings, based on changing needs and available resources

Continuum of care – conceptual model that describes a person's movement from wellness through desired quality of life to dignified death. A person's place on the continuum is determined individually.

Criteria – relevant, measurable indicators of the standards of clinical nursing practice

Critical care nurse – licensed professional nurse who provides direct care or influences care for acutely/critically ill or injured patients who are at high risk for actual or potential life-threatening health problems, regardless of the work setting for their nursing care[8]

Cultural humility – includes a process of self-reflection and discovery to challenge one's own cultural biases and build a humble and respectful attitude toward individuals of other cultures[9]

Culturally safe – reflective process that enables nurses to provide safe patient care that is defined by those who receive the care[10]

CUS – Concerned, Uncomfortable, and Safety/Stop. A mnemonic that provides a tool for advocacy, assertion, and mutual support to improve patient safety and bring awareness to a potential issue that could cause harm. CUS is also a recommended tool to express concerns regarding the need for a medical interpreter when conversations involve patients with limited English proficiency.[11]

De-escalation – combination of strategies, techniques, and methods used with the goal of reducing a patient's agitation and aggression. Examples include communication, self-regulation, assessment, actions, and safety maintenance in order to reduce the risk of harm to patients and caregivers as well as the use of restraints or seclusion.[12]

Diagnosis – clinical judgment on the patient's response to actual or potential health conditions or needs. It may be a medical or nursing diagnosis and provides the basis for determining an interprofessional plan of care to achieve expected outcomes.

Direct care time – time directly associated with patient care or performance of nursing tasks; sometimes referred to as productive time. The opposite is sometimes referred to as nonproductive time or indirect care time, which is the time required to assess, plan, and evaluate care, as well as time spent on education and committee work.[13]

Disaster – serious disruption in the functioning of a community or society on any scale due to hazardous events interacting with conditions of exposure, vulnerability, and capacity, leading to 1 or more of the following: human, material, economic, and environmental losses and impacts[14]

Diversity (encompasses culture, gender, sex, ethics, etc) – state or fact of being diverse; difference; unlikeness. Diversity goes well beyond race, ethnicity, gender, disability status, and age; it encompasses mutable characteristics such as education and immutable characteristics such as birth order.[15]

End-of-life care – patient care before death, either while undergoing curative treatment or after deciding to focus on comfort rather than cure[16]

Engagement – the employee's emotional commitment to the organization and its goals[17]

Environment of care – made up of 3 basic elements. The arrangement of the building or space and the features that protect patients, visitors, and staff. The equipment used to support patient care or to safely operate the building or space. The people who work in the hospital, the patients, and all who enter the environment[18]

Equity, diversity, and inclusion (EDI)

- Equity recognizes differences and actively provides all people with the necessary resources and fair opportunities to attain their full potential.
- Diversity includes the spectrum of individual differences, identities, cultures, and group memberships that human beings have in society. Embracing diversity respects values and celebrates the many aspects of being human.
- Inclusion is the active, intentional, ongoing engagement with diversity, including intentional policies and practices promoting full participation and a feeling of belonging. Inclusion acknowledges challenges faced and values the collaborative contributions of lived differences. It requires acknowledgment of unconscious bias.[19]

Escalation – awareness of the different types of physical and nonphysical acts and threats of workplace violence and signs that these acts may increase[20]

Evaluation – process of determining the patient's progress toward attainment of expected outcomes

Evidence and levels: AACN's evidence-leveling system[21]

AACN Levels of Evidence

Level A Meta-analysis of quantitative studies or metasynthesis of qualitative studies with results that consistently support a specific action, intervention, or treatment (including systematic review of randomized controlled trials)

Level B Well-designed, controlled studies with results that consistently support a specific action, intervention, or treatment

Level C Qualitative studies, descriptive or correlational studies, integrative reviews, systematic reviews, or randomized controlled trials with inconsistent results

Level D Peer-reviewed professional and organizational standards with the support of clinical study recommendations

Level E Multiple case reports, theory-based evidence from expert opinions, or peer-reviewed professional organizational standards without clinical studies to support recommendations

Level M Manufacturer's recommendations only

Evidence-based practice (EBP) – a problem-solving approach to practice that involves the conscientious use of current best evidence in making decisions about patient care. EBP incorporates a systematic search for and critical appraisal of the most relevant evidence to answer a clinical question, along with one's clinical expertise and the patient's values and preferences.[22]

Family – family of origin, chosen family, and/or significant others, as identified by the patient

Fiduciary – legal or ethical relationship of trust with 1 or more other parties[23]

Financial stewardship/contribution – performance improvements that enhance patient safety and resource stewardship for positive outcomes, reducing the cost of care

Guidelines – clinical practice guidelines or statements that include recommendations intended to optimize patient care. They are informed by a systematic review of evidence and an assessment of the benefits and harms of alternative care options.[24]

Healing, humane, and caring environment – progressive care nurses practice in settings with patients requiring complex assessments and interventions. Nursing is a constant in the progressive care environment. As part of an interprofessional team, nurses work to create healing, humane, and caring environments in which:

- Providers act as advocates on behalf of patients, families, and communities
- Patient and family values dominate
- Ethical decision making is supported, fostered, and promoted

As part of an interprofessional team, nurses work to create healing, humane, and caring environments in which: (Cont'd)

- Collaboration is embraced
- Leadership is fostered at all levels and in all activities
- Lifelong learning is fundamental to professional growth
- Existing talents and resources are optimized
- Innovation and creativity are rewarded
- Diversity is respected

Health care providers – individuals with special expertise who provide health care services or assistance to patients: including nurses, advanced practice nurses, physicians, psychologists, social workers, nutritionists, dieticians, and various therapists

Health data – collection of information related to the health, reproductive outcomes, life span, causes of death, and/or quality outcomes for a patient or population[25]

Health data equity – health systems data repositories that are a true reflection of patient's life experiences. The goal is to have equitable data that will address health care inequities.[26,27]

Health equity – a state in which everyone has a fair and just opportunity to attain their highest level of health. Achieving this state requires focused and ongoing societal efforts to address historical and contemporary injustices; overcome economic, social, and other obstacles to health and health care; and eliminate preventable health disparities.[27]

Health literacy – degree to which individuals have the ability to find, understand, interpret, and use information and services to inform health-related decisions and actions for themselves and others[28]

Healthy work environment – work environments that are safe, healing, humane, and respectful of the rights, responsibilities, needs, and contributions of all people – including patients, their families, nurses, and other health care professionals. It is a work environment that supports the standards of skilled communication, true collaboration, effective decision making, appropriate staffing, meaningful recognition, and authentic leadership.[29]

Holistic – considering all aspects of an individual or population's health[30]

Implementation – process of carrying out the interprofessional plan of care, which may include implementing, delegating, and/or coordinating interventions. The patient, and/or family, or health care providers may be designated to implement interventions in the plan.

Implicit or unconscious bias – social stereotypes about certain groups of people that individuals form outside their own conscious awareness. Individuals' perceptions and behaviors can be influenced by the implicit biases they hold, even if they are unaware they hold such biases. Implicit bias is an aspect of implicit social cognition: the phenomenon that perceptions, attitudes, and stereotypes can operate prior to conscious intention or endorsement.[31]

Incivility – discourteous, rude, or disrespectful behavior or treatment

Indirect care time – sometimes referred to as nonproductive or administrative time; not directly associated with patient care or performance of nursing tasks. It is the time required to assess, plan, and evaluate care, as well as time spent on education and committee work. The opposite is referred to as direct care time, also referred to as productive time, which is directly associated with patient care or performance of nursing tasks.[13]

Intellectual disability – significant impairment in intellectual ability accompanied by deficits in skills necessary for independent daily functioning[32]

Judgment – formation of a conclusion that encompasses critical thinking, problem solving, ethical reasoning, and decision making

Just culture – a culture where all team members have a shared responsibility and accountability for fairness and response to safety issues and foster an open work culture[33]

Legal guardian – a person who has the legal authority to care for the personal and property interests of an incapacitated senior, a minor, or a developmentally disabled adult[34]

Moral distress – presence of constraints, either internal (personal) or external (institutional) that prevent one from taking actions that one perceives to be morally right[35]

Nonproductive time – time not directly associated with patient care or performance of nursing tasks. Time required to assess, plan, and evaluate care, as well as time spent on education and committee work. Sometimes referred to as indirect care time[13]

Nurse – an individual who is licensed by a state agency to practice as a registered nurse

Nurse competencies (from the AACN Synergy Model)[2] – reflect an integration of knowledge, skills, experience, and attitudes needed to meet the needs of patients and families. The continuum of nurse competencies, which is derived from patient needs, is composed of the following:

- Clinical judgment – clinical reasoning, which includes clinical decision making, critical thinking, and a global grasp of the situation, coupled with nursing skills acquired through a process of integrating formal and informal experiential knowledge and evidence-based guidelines
- Advocacy and moral agency – working on another's behalf and representing the concerns of the patient, family, and community; serving as a moral agent in identifying and helping to resolve ethical and clinical concerns in the clinical setting
- Caring practices – constellation of nursing activities that are responsive to the uniqueness of the patient and family and create a compassionate and therapeutic environment, with the aim of promoting comfort and preventing suffering. These caring behaviors include, but are not limited to, vigilance, engagement, and responsiveness.

- Collaboration – working with others (eg, patients, families, and health care providers) in a way that promotes and encourages each person's contribution toward achieving optimal and realistic patient goals. Collaboration involves intra- and interprofessional work with all colleagues.
- Systems thinking – body of knowledge and tools that allow nurses to appreciate the care environment from a perspective that recognizes the holistic interrelationship within and across health care systems
- Responses to diversity – the sensitivity to recognize, appreciate, and incorporate differences in the provision of care. Differences involving patients, families, and members of the health care team may include, but are not limited to, individuality, cultural differences (eg, regarding child rearing, family relations), spiritual beliefs, gender, race, ethnicity, disability, family configuration, lifestyle, socioeconomic status, age, values, and alternative medicine.
- Facilitation of learning – ability to facilitate learning for patients/families, nursing staff, other members of the health care team, and community. Includes both formal and informal facilitation of learning
- Clinical inquiry or innovator/evaluator – ongoing process of questioning and evaluating practice, providing informed practice, and innovating through research and experiential learning. The nurse engages in clinical knowledge development to promote the best patient outcomes.

Nursing – health care profession that protects, promotes, and optimizes patient health and abilities, prevents illness and injury, alleviates suffering through the diagnosis and treatment of human responses, and provides advocacy in the care of patients, families, communities, and populations[36]

Nursing process – dynamic, systematic method of caring for patients from a nursing perspective. The stages of the nursing process are assessment, diagnosis, outcomes identification, planning, implementation, and evaluation. The dynamic and circular nature of the nursing process is apparent in the nurse's continual collection (recollection) and assessment (reassessment) of data, the patient's response to care, formulation (reformulation) of the outcomes to be expected, and provision of interventions based on these data. The circular nature of the nursing process assumes that nurses include the patient, family, and health care team in the formulation of the plan. The nursing process forms the foundation of the nurse's decision making.[37]

Outcomes – measurable, expected goals. Agency for Healthcare Research and Quality defines outcomes as the impact of a health care service or intervention and can include these events or result in:

- Patient health status or quality of life
- Patient, provider, and population attitudes and behavior
- New evidence, research, prevention strategies, treatments, and care models[38]

The term *expected outcomes* describes the results that are anticipated, measurable, desirable, equitable and observable, and translate into observable behaviors as a result of the interventions of the nurse and other members of the interdisciplinary team.[37]

Palliative care – improves the quality of life of patients (adults and children) and their families who are facing problems associated with life-threatening illnesses. It prevents and relieves suffering through the early identification, correct assessment, and management of pain and other problems, whether physical, psychosocial, or spiritual.[39]

Patient – recipient of nursing care. The term patient is used here to provide consistency and brevity, bearing in mind that the term *patient* or the term *individual* might be a better choice in some instances. When the patient is an individual, the focus is on the health state, problems, or needs of a single person. When the patient is a family or group, the focus is on the health state of the whole or the reciprocal effects of an individual's health state on other members of the group. When the patient is a community, the focus is on the personal and environmental health and health risks of population groups. Patients can be described by a number of characteristics. All characteristics are connected and contribute to each other.

Patient characteristics (from the AACN Synergy Model[2]) span the continuum of health and illness:

- Resiliency – capacity to return to a restorative level of functioning using compensatory coping mechanisms; ability to bounce back quickly after an insult
- Vulnerability – susceptibility to actual or potential stressors that may adversely affect patient outcomes
- Stability – ability to maintain steady-state equilibrium
- Complexity – intricate entanglement of 2 or more systems (eg, body, family, therapies)
- Resource availability – extent of resources (eg, technical, fiscal, personal, psychological, social) that the patient, family, and community bring to the situation
- Participation in care – extent to which the patient and family engage in aspects of care
- Participation in decision making – extent to which the patient and family engage in decision making
- Predictability – a summative characteristic that allows one to expect a certain course of events or course of illness

Patient/family – *Patient* refers to an individual person, while *family* can include the family of origin, chosen family, or significant others as identified by the patient. The term patient/family provides consistency and brevity in the focus of the services of the progressive care nurse.

Peer review – process by which professionals with similar KSAs judge the processes and/or outcomes of care

Plan of care – interprofessional outline of care based on expected outcomes for a particular patient. The patient, family, and health care providers participate in carrying out the plan for the implementation or delivery of care.

Practice analysis – also known as a job analysis or role delineation study: any of several methods used singly or in combination to identify the performance domains and associated tasks, knowledge, and/or skills related to the purpose of the credential and to provide the foundation for certification exam validation. The analysis helps identify the tasks and work activities conducted, the context in which those tasks and activities are carried out, and the competencies (knowledge areas, skills, and abilities) required to perform a role successfully.[40]

Prescribe – advise and authorize the use of a medication or treatment[41]

Privacy – The nurse's duty to maintain confidentiality is foundational to the ethical obligation to respect individuals' dignity and autonomy and the patient's right to protection of their health care information.[42]

Professional identity – defined as a sense of oneself, and in relationship with others, that is influenced by characteristics, norms, and values of the nursing discipline, resulting in an individual feeling, thinking, and acting as a nurse[37]

Professional opportunities – participating in advocacy, research, professional organizations, professional development, practice innovations, advanced degrees, specialty certification, publishing, media engagement, content creation, mentoring, leadership development, etc

Professional values – attitudes and behaviors that inform and direct a nurse's decision-making process. Can be formed over time and influenced by culture, education, family, and the environment[37]

Progressive care – location of acutely ill adult patients who are moderately stable with an elevated risk of instability. These patients require a high intensity of care and vigilance.[43]

Progressive care nurse – licensed professional nurse who provides direct care or influences care for acutely ill patients who are moderately stable with an elevated risk of instability. These patients require a high intensity of care and vigilance.[43]

Progressive care nursing – specialty within nursing that deals specifically with human responses to actual or potential life-threatening health symptoms and diagnoses.[43]

Psychologically safe – Psychological safety results in the shared belief that someone will not be rejected or humiliated for speaking up with ideas, questions, concerns, or mistakes.[44]

Quality of care – cooperative and collaborative process that combines the goals of professional standards of care with the defined expectations of the patient and family

Reflective practice – ability to reflect on one's actions through a recurrent thoughtful and personal self-assessment, analysis, and synthesis of strengths and opportunities for improvement[45]

Resilience – process of adapting positively in the face of adversity, trauma, tragedy, threats, or significant stress[46]

Self-care – practice of taking action to preserve or improve one's health

Self-determination – ability to make choices and manage life, including a nurse managing their professional life[37]

Shared decision making – model of care that engages patients in making choices about their care. Patients actively work with a nurse or other health care professionals to make informed decisions about their health care options.[47]

Skill – an ability with psychomotor, communication, interpersonal, and diagnostic components

Skilled communication – Nurses must be as proficient in communication skills as they are in clinical skills. According to the American Association of Critical-Care Nurses, there are 5 critical elements for organizations and 8 critical elements for nurses.[48]

Staffing – effective match between patient needs and nurse competencies

Standard – authoritative statement, articulated and supported by the profession, that describes a level of care or performance by which the quality of practice, service, or education can be measured or judged

Standards of care – authoritative statements that describe a competent level of clinical nursing practice demonstrated through assessment, diagnosis, outcome identification, planning, implementation, and evaluation

Standards of practice – authoritative statements that describe a level of care or performance common to the profession of nursing and by which the quality of nursing practices can be judged. Standards of clinical nursing practice include standards of care and standards of professional performance.

Standards of professional performance – authoritative statements that describe a competent level of behavior in a professional role, including activities related to quality of care, performance appraisal, education, collegiality, ethics, collaboration, research, resource utilization, and leadership

Surrogate – one appointed to act in place of another[49]

Telehealth – connects individuals and their health care providers when in-person care is not necessary or not possible in order to improve patients' health status. The American Telemedicine Association views telemedicine and telehealth as interchangeable terms.[51]

TeleICU/tele-critical care – collaborative interprofessional care model focusing on assessment, evaluation, surveillance, and other nursing activities of critically ill patients that is enabled by leveraging audio, video, data, and other technologies to engage care experts in patient care, partnered with clinicians at collaborating sites. Services may be expanded to include other acutely ill patients at a high risk for instability.[50]

Transitions of care – process of transferring a patient's care from 1 setting or level of care to another, such as from progressive care to critical care, hospital to home, or hospital to skilled nursing facility. These transitions are particularly vulnerable points in the health care continuum.[52]

Unconscious bias – See implicit bias.

Virtual nursing – delivery of patient care and services from a remote location. It supplements care provided to patients and reduces the burden on direct care nurses.[53]

Work-life balance – amount of time spent doing one's job compared with the amount of time spent with family and friends or on activities outside of work[54]

Workplace violence – threat of violence against workers. It can occur within or outside the workplace and can range from threats and verbal abuse to physical assaults and homicide[55,56]

Zero tolerance – law, policy, or practice that provides severe penalties for a proscribed offense or behavior without making exceptions

REFERENCES

1. American Association of Critical-Care Nurses. AACN core values. Accessed August 1, 2024. https://www.aacn.org/about-aacn

2. AACN Certification Corporation. AACN Synergy Model for Patient Care. Accessed August 13, 2024. http://www.aacn.org/wd/certifications/content/synmodel.pcms?menu=certification

3. Jennings BM. Chapter 23: Patient acuity. In Hughes RG ed. *Patient Safety and Quality: An Evidence-Based Handbook for Nurses.* Accessed August 1, 2024. https://www.ncbi.nlm.nih.gov/books/NBK2680/

4. Moss, M, Good VS, Gozal D, et al. An official Critical Care Societies Collaborative statement: burnout syndrome in critical care health care professionals: A call for action. *Am J Crit Care.* 2016;25(4):368–376.

5. Wikipedia. Caregiver. Accessed August 1, 2024. https://en.wikipedia.org/wiki/Caregiver

6. American Nurses Association. Professional role competence. Accessed March 5, 2019. https://www.nursingworld.org/practice-policy/nursing-excellence/official-position-statements/id/professional-role-competence/

7. Alspach JG. *Designing Competency Assessment Programs: A Handbook for Nursing and Health-Related Professions.* National Nursing Staff Development Organization; 1995.

8. AACN Certification Corporation. A job analysis of the acute/critical care nurse. AACN Certification Corporation; 2018.

9. Yeager KA, Bauer-Wu S. Cultural humility: essential foundation for clinical researchers. *Appl Nurs Res.* 2013;26(4). Accessed August 1, 2024. doi:10.1016/j.apnr.2013.06.008

10. Curtis E, Jones R, Tipene-Leach D, et al. Why cultural safety rather than cultural competency is required to achieve health equity: a literature review and recommended definition. *Int J Equity Health.* 2019;18(174). Accessed August 1, 2024. https://doi.org/10.1186/s12939-019-1082-3

11. Agency for Healthcare Research and Quality. Tool: CUS. Accessed August 6, 2024. https://www.ahrq.gov/teamstepps-program/curriculum/mutual/tools/cus.html

12. The Joint Commission. De-escalation in health care. Accessed August 1, 2024. https://www.jointcommission.org/-/media/tjc/documents/resources/workplace-violence/qs_deescalation_1_28_18_final.pdf

13. Altman M, Rosa W. Redefining "time" to meet nursing's evolving demands. *Nurs Crit Care.* 2018;11(3):12–15. https://journals.lww.com/nursing/abstract/2016/03000/redefining__time__to_meet_nursing_s_evolving.16.aspx

14. PreventionWeb. Terminology: disaster. Accessed August 1, 2024. https://www.preventionweb.net/terminology/view/475

15. Office of Diversity and Inclusion. US Department of Veterans Affairs. Glossary of terms. Accessed August 1, 2024. https://www.diversity.va.gov/tools/glossary.aspx

16. American Association of Critical-Care Nurses. Palliative care in acute & critical care settings. Accessed August 1, 2024. https://www.aacn.org/clinical-resources/palliative-end-of-life

17. Kruse K. What is employee engagement? *Forbes*. June 22, 2012. Accessed August 1, 2024. https://www.forbes.com/sites/kevinkruse/2012/06/22/employee-engagement-what-and-why/#788e49b07f37

18. The Joint Commission. Environment of care. Accessed August 2, 2024. https://www.jointcommission.org/standards/standard-faqs/hospital-and-hospital-clinics/environment-of-care-ec/000001284/

19. American Association of Critical-Care Nurses. AACN EDI Community Network. Equity, diversity and inclusion definitions. Accessed August 2, 2024.

20. Dictionary.com. Adapted definition of escalation. Accessed August 1, 2024.

21. Peterson MH, Barnason S, Donnelly B, et al. Choosing the best evidence to guide clinical practice: application of AACN levels of evidence. *Crit Care Nurse.* 2014;34(2):58–68. https://aacnjournals.org/ccnonline/article/34/2/58/3284/Choosing-the-Best-Evidence-to-Guide-Clinical

22. Melnyk BM, Fineout-Overholt E. *Evidence-Based Practice in Nursing & Healthcare: A Guide to Best Practice.* Lippincott Williams & Wilkins; 2005:387.

23. Wikipedia. Fiduciary. Accessed August 1, 2024. https://en.wikipedia.org/wiki/Fiduciary

24. Institute of Medicine (US) Committee on Standards for Developing Trustworthy Clinical Practice Guidelines; Graham R, Mancher M, Miller Wolman D, et al, eds. *Clinical Practice Guidelines We Can Trust.* National Academies Press; 2011:1. Accessed March 5, 2019. https://www.ncbi.nlm.nih.gov/books/NBK209546/

25. Wikipedia. Health data. Accessed August 1, 2024. https://en.wikipedia.org/wiki/Health_data

26. Robert Wood Johnson Foundation. Charting a course for an equity-centered data system. Accessed August 1, 2024. https://www.rwjf.org/en/insights/our-research/2021/10/charting-a-course-for-an-equity-centered-data-system.html

27. CDC Foundation. Principles for using public health data to drive equity: a guide to embedding equitable practices throughout the data life cycle. Accessed August 1, 2024. https://www.cdcfoundation.org/data-equity-principles?inline

28. Healthy People 2030. Health literacy in healthy people 2030. Accessed August 1, 2024. https://health.gov/healthypeople/priority-areas/health-literacy-healthy-people-2030

29. Barden C, ed. *AACN Standards for Establishing and Sustaining Healthy Work Environments: A Journey to Excellence.* 2nd ed. American Association of Critical-Care Nurses; 2016:9.

30. Mosby's Dictionary of Medicine, Nursing & Health Professions. Holistic.

31. American Psychological Association. Implicit bias. Accessed August 2, 2024. https://www.apa.org/topics/implicit-bias

32. American Association on Intellectual and Developmental Disabilities. Frequently asked questions on intellectual disability. Accessed August 1, 2024. https://www.aaidd.org/intellectual-disability/faqs-on-intellectual-disability

33. Robichaux C, Vittone S. Ethics: addressing error: partnership in a just culture. *OJIN.* April 25, 2023. Accessed August 1, 2024. https://doi.org/10.3912/OJIN.Vol28No02EthCol01

34. Wikipedia. Legal guardian. Accessed August 1, 2024. https://en.wikipedia.org/wiki/Legal_guardian

35. Hamric AB, Davis W, Childress MD. Moral distress in health-care providers: what is it and what can we do about it? *Pharos Alpha Omega Alpha Honor Med Soc.* 2006;69:16–23.

36. American Nurses Association. *Nursing's Social Policy Statement: The Essence of the Profession.* Nursesbooks.org; 2010.

37. American Nurses Association. *Nursing: Scope and Standards of Practice.* 4th ed. Nursingworld.org; 2021.

38. Agency for Healthcare Research and Quality. Topic: outcomes. Accessed August 5, 2024. https://www.ahrq.gov/topics/outcomes.html

39. World Health Organization. Palliative care. Accessed August 5, 2024. https://www.who.int/news-room/fact-sheets/detail/palliative-care

40. I.C.E. Terminology Taskforce. *Basic Guide to Credentialing Terminology.* 2nd ed. Institute for Credentialing Excellence; 2020.

41. Oxford English Dictionary. Prescribe. Accessed March 5, 2019. https://en.oxforddictionaries.com/definition/prescribe

42. ANA Center for Ethics and Human Rights. Privacy and confidentiality. Accessed August 5, 2024. https://www.nursingworld.org/practice-policy/nursing-excellence/official-position-statements/id/privacy-and-confidentiality/

43. AACN Certification Corporation. A job analysis of the progressive care nurse. AACN Certification Corporation; 2023.

44. American Association of Critical-Care Nurses. EDI Community Network Intranet Page. Accessed August 5, 2024.

45. Wikipedia. Reflective practice. Accessed August 5, 2024. https://en.wikipedia.org/wiki/Reflective_practice

46. American Psychological Association. Resilience. Accessed September 16, 2024. https://www.apa.org/topics/resilience

47. Skelly CL, Hall CA, Risher CR. Shared decision making and patient-centered care. *Am Nurse.* 2020. Accessed August 5, 2024. https://www.myamericannurse.com/shared-decision-making-and-patient-centered-care/

48. American Association of Critical-Care Nurses. Skilled communication. Accessed August 5, 2024. https://www.aacn.org/nursing-excellence/healthy-work-environments/skilled-communication

49. Merriam-Webster. Surrogate. Accessed August 5, 2024. https://www.merriam-webster.com/dictionary/surrogate

50. American Association of Critical-Care Nurses. *AACN Tele-critical Care Nursing Practice: An Expert Consensus Statement Supporting Acute, Progressive and Critical Care 2022.* Accessed August 5, 2024. https://www.aacn.org/nursing-excellence/standards/aacn-tele-critical-care-nursing-consensus-statement

51. American Telemedicine Association. Telehealth: defining 21st century care. https://www.americantelemed.org/resource/why-telemedicine/

52. Transitions of Care. Transitions of care standards. Accessed August 5, 2024. https://transitionsofcare.org/

53. Advisory Board. Virtual nursing: what it is and why we need it. Accessed August 5, 2024. https://www.advisory.com/content/dam/advisory/en/public/success-pages/virtual-nursing-cheat-sheet.pdf.coredownload.pdf

54. Schwartz SP, Adair KC, Bae J, et al. Work-life balance behaviours cluster in work settings and relate to burnout and safety culture: a cross-sectional survey analysis [published online October 11, 2018]. *BMJ Qual Saf.* doi:10.1136/bmjqs-2018-007933

55. US Department of Labor. Occupational Safety and Health Administration. Healthcare wide hazards: workplace violence. Accessed August 5, 2024. https://www.osha.gov/SLTC/etools/hospital/hazards/workplaceviolence/viol.html

56. US Department of Labor. Occupational Safety and Health Administration. Workplace violence. Accessed August 5, 2024. https://www.osha.gov/SLTC/workplaceviolence/

APPENDIX

Resources to Support Implementation of *AACN Scope and Standards for Progressive Care Nursing Practice*

AACN Resources

Scope of Practice

- Hartigan C. Scope of practice. *Crit Care Nurse.* 2016;36(5):70–72. Accessed March 5, 2019. http://ccn.aacnjournals.org/content/36/5/70.full

Nurse Staffing

- *AACN Standards for Appropriate Staffing in Adult Critical Care* https://www.aacn.org/nursing-excellence/standards/aacn-standards-for-appropriate-staffing-in-adult-critical-care
- Protecting Your Nursing License When Staffing Is Suboptimal https://www.aacn.org/blog/protecting-your-nursing-license-when-staffing-is-suboptimal
- Nurse Staffing: Ratios, Reimbursement and the Work Environment https://www.aacn.org/blog/nurse-staffing-ratios-reimbursement-and-the-work-environment

Development of Competence for Progressive Care Nursing

- AACN Orientation Pathway https://www.aacn.org/education/new-nurse-orientation?tab=Single-Site%20LearnCenter
    - AACN New Nurse Online Community https://aacn.mobilize.io/registrations/groups/64856
    - AACN Knowledge Assessment Tool for Entry Level Progressive Care Nursing https://www.aacn.org/education/knowledge-assessment-tool
    - AACN Essentials of Critical Care Orientation = Progressive Care Track https://www.aacn.org/education/online-courses/essentials-of-critical-care-orientation?tab=Successful%20Completion
    - AACN Competence Framework & Toolkit https://www.aacn.org/education/competence-framework-toolkit

Communities for Professional Networking and Engagement

- AACN Communities https://www.aacn.org/clinical-resources/online-nursing-community-forums

Nurse Well-Being and the Work Environment

- AACN Healthy Work Environment Standards https://www.aacn.org/nursing-excellence/healthy-work-environments

APPENDIX

Nurse Well-Being and the Work Environment (Cont'd)

- AACN Healthy Work Environment Assessment Tools https://www.aacn.org/nursing-excellence/healthy-work-environments#assessments
- Moral Distress Web Page https://www.aacn.org/clinical-resources/moral-distress
- Peer Support Community - available to AACN members only https://www.aacn.org/clinical-resources/online-nursing-community-forums
- Support for the Second Victim: Caring for Our Own https://www.aacn.org/education/ce-activities/wb0039/support-for-the-second-victim-caring-for-our-own
- Second Victim: Supporting the Error-Maker in the ICU https://www.aacn.org/education/ce-activities/nti22266/second-victim-supporting-the-errormaker-in-the-icu
- Suicide: A Dark Cloud Over Nursing https://www.aacn.org/blog/suicide-a-dark-cloud-over-nursing
- Suicide Among Nurses: We have to talk about it https://www.aacn.org/blog/suicide-among-nurses-we-have-to-talk-about-it
- The Impact of Nurses' Work Environment on Mental Health and Suicide https://www.aacn.org/education/publications/ccn/44/3/0006-guest-editorial-the-impact-of-nurses-work-environment-on-mental-health-and-suicide

Professionalism in Nursing

- Do's and Don'ts of Social Media Use for Nursing Professionals https://www.aacn.org/blog/dos-and-donts-of-social-media-use-for-nursing-professionals
- Two Questions That Educators Should Ask All New Nurses https://www.aacn.org/blog/two-questions-that-educators-should-ask-all-new-nurses
- Can I Do That? Incorporating the Scope and Standards of Practice Into Nursing Professional Development https://www.aacn.org/blog/can-i-do-that-incorporating-scope-and-standards-of-practice-into-nursing-professional-development

Professional Resource

- Call to Action: Blueprint for Change in Acute and Critical CareNursing. *Nurs Outlook.* 2024;72(6):1–10. Accessed September 16, 2024. https://www.sciencedirect.com/science/article/pii/S0029655424001647

AMERICAN
ASSOCIATION
of CRITICAL-CARE
NURSES

Made in the USA
Monee, IL
13 September 2026

62981005R00057